Serono Symposia Publications from Raven Press
Volume 1

Luminescent Assays
Perspectives in Endocrinology and Clinical Chemistry

Serono Symposia Publications from Raven Press
Volume 1

Luminescent Assays
Perspectives in Endocrinology and Clinical Chemistry

Editors

Mario Serio
Chair of Endocrinology
University of Sassari
Sassari, Italy

Mario Pazzagli
Endocrinology Unit
University of Florence
Florence, Italy

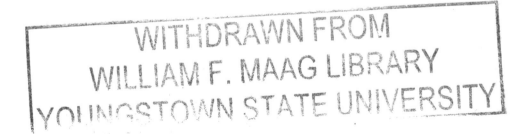

Raven Press ■ New York

Raven Press, 1140 Avenue of the Americas, New York, New York 10036

Made in the United States of America

International Standard Book Number 0-89004-740-5
Library of Congress Catalog Number 81-40363

Preface

Luminescent assays are new promising techniques in the field of clinical chemistry with a wide range of practical applications in Medicine and Biology. Luminescent labels, in relation to high sensitivity, represent a new and realistic alternative to radioactive labels for measurements of hormones in biological fluid by competitive binding assays.

This volume provides a comprehensive review of luminescent assays and their applications to human function. Topics include basic aspects of luminescent systems and instrumentations, applications of firefly luciferase, analytical applications of bacterial luminescent system, assays using bioluminescence in clinical chemistry and endocrinology, chemiluminescent systems for measurement of steroids and polipeptide hormones, chemiluminescence assays in the diagnosis of immuno and hematological diseases.

This book will be of interest to biologists, endocrinologists, immunologists, hematologists, and other researchers involved in a variety of areas of clinical chemistry.

Mario Serio
Mario Pazzagli

Acknowledgments

The chapters in this volume summarize lectures presented at the Meeting on Luminescent Assays: Perspectives in Endocrinology and Clinical Chemistry, held in Florence in July 1981 and organized by the Post-Graduate School of Endocrinology of the University of Florence in collaboration with the Serono Symposia.

This Meeting would not have taken place without the dedicated efforts of a number of people. In particular we are grateful to the members of the Scientific Committee Prof. V. H. T. James (U. K.), Prof. H. R. Lindner (Israel), Prof. E. Schram (Belgium), Prof. A. Borghi, Prof. E. Ferroni, Prof. G. Giusti, Prof. L. Martini, and Prof. F. Pasquinelli (Italy), who brought together a group of very distinguished speakers who provided a comprehensive, authoritative, and up-to-date overview of the field.

The scientific efforts would have been of little avail without the very generous financial support of Serono Symposia, Region of Tuscany, Province of Florence and City of Florence.

A special acknowledgment must go to the staff of the Organizzazione Internazionale Congressi, Florence, for its interest in the Meeting and valuable help with its organization.

Contents

Contributors

E. Albert
Immunogenetics Laboratory
Kinderpoliklinik der Universität
8000 Munich, Federal Republic of Germany

Robert C. Allen
Department of Clinical Investigation and
U.S. Army Institute of Surgical Research
Brooke Army Medical Center
Fort Sam Houston, Texas 78234

L. Altomonte
Department of Internal Medicine
Università Cattolica S. Cuore
00168 Rome, Italy

K. Bergström
Department of Clinical Chemistry
Karolinska Institute
Huddinge Hospital
S-141 86 Huddinge, Sweden

Fritz Berthold
Laboratorium Professor Dr. Berthold
P.O. Box 160
D-7547 Wildbad, Federal Republic of Germany

G. F. Bolelli
Physiopathology of Reproduction Service
University of Bologna
Bologna, Italy

R. Botti
ISVT Sclavo
Research Center
53100 Siena, Italy

S. E. Brolin
Department of Medical Cell Biology
University of Uppsala
Biomedicum, Box 571
S-751 23 Uppsala, Sweden

David G. Burleson
Department of Clinical Investigation and
U.S. Army Institute of Surgical Research
Brooke Army Medical Center
Fort Sam Houston, Texas 78234

U. Busch
Immunogenetics Laboratory
Kinderpoliklinik der Universität
8000 Munich, Federal Republic of Germany

A. L. Caldini
Endocrinology Unit
University of Florence
Viale Morgagni 85
50134 Florence, Italy

A. K. Campbell
Department of Medical Biochemistry
Welsh National School of Medicine
Heath Park
Cardiff CP4 4XN, United Kingdom

W. P. Collins
Department of Obstetrics and Gynaecology
King's College Hospital Medical School
Denmark Hill
London SE5 8RX, Great Britain

F. Comhaire
Department of Internal Medicine
State University of Ghent
Academisch Ziekenhuis
De Pintelaan 135
B-9000 Ghent, Belgium

S. Cuomo
Endocrinology Unit
University of Florence
Viale Morgagni 83
50134 Florence, Italy

Marlene DeLuca
Department of Chemistry
University of California at San Diego
La Jolla, California 92093

P. De Sole
Institute of Biological Chemistry
Università Cattolica S. Cuore
00168 Rome, Italy

H. Egghart
Mobility Equipment Research and Development
Command
Fort Belvoir, Virginia 22060

M. Ernst
Max-Planck-Institut für Immunbiologie
Freiburg, Federal Republic of Germany

Th. M. Ernst
Haut- und Poliklinik der Freien Universität
  Berlin im Rudolf Virchow-Krankenhaus
  Augustenburger Platz 1
D-1000 Berlin 65, West Germany

Z. Eshhar
Department of Chemical Immunology
The Weizmann Institute of Science
P.O. Box 26
Rehovot 76100, Israel

S. Falkenberg
Robert Koch-Institute des
  Bundesgesundheitsamtes
Nordufer 20
D-1000 Berlin 65, West Germany

G. Fiorelli
Endocrinology Unit
University of Florence
Viale Morgagni 85
50134 Florence, Italy

H. Fischer
Max-Planck-Institut für Immunbiologie
Freiburg, Federal Republic of Germany

G. Ghirlanda
Department of Internal Medicine
Università Cattolica S. Cuore
00168 Roma, Italy

K.-E. Gillert
Robert Koch-Institut des
  Bundesgesundheitsamtes
Nordufer 20
D-1000 Berlin 65, West Germany

A. V. Greco
Department of Internal Medicine
Università Cattolica S. Cuore
00168 Rome, Italy

K.D. Gundermann
Organisch-Chemisches Institut
Technische Universität Clausthal
3392 Clausthal-Zellerfeld, Federal Republic of
  Germany

Hans-Peter Haar
Boehringer Mannheim GmbH
Research Center Tutzing
D-8132 Tutzing, Federal Republic of Germany

R. C. Hart
School of Molecular Sciences
Sussex University
Palmer
Sussex, United Kingdom

M. Heberer
Kantonsspital
Basel, Switzerland

H. Kather
Klinisches Institut für Herzinfarktforschung
Medizinische Universitätsklinik
Bergheimer Strasse 58
D-6900 Heidelberg, West Germany

T. Kato
Universitätshautklinik
Freiburg, Federal Republic of Germany

J. B. Kim
Department of Hormone Research
The Weizmann Institute of Science
P.O. Box 26
Rehovot 76100, Israel and
Department of Obstetrics and Gynaecology
King's College Hospital Medical School
Denmark Hill
London SE5 8RX, Great Britain

Ahuva Knysznski
Department of Membrane Research
The Weizmann Institute of Science
Rehovot 76100, Israel

F. Kohen
Department of Hormone Research
The Weizmann Institute of Science
P.O. Box 26
Rehovot 76100, Israel

Larry J. Kricka
Department of Clinical Chemistry
Wolfson Research Laboratories
University of Birmingham
Birgmingham B15 2TH, United Kingdom

Helmut Kubisiak
Laboratorium Professor Dr. Berthold
P.O. Box 160
D-7547 Wildbad, Federal Republic of Germany

P. Leoncini
ISVT Sclavo
Research Center
53100 Siena, Italy

H. R. Lindner
Department of Hormone Research
The Weizmann Institute of Science
P.O. Box 26
Rehovot 76100, Israel

R. Linke
Boehringer Mannheim GmbH
Research Center Tutzing
P.O. Box 120
8132 Tutzing, Federal Republic of Germany

S. Lippa
Institute of Biological Chemistry
Università Cattolica S. Cuore
00168 Rome, Italy

Richard D. Lippman
Department of Medical Cell Biology
University of Uppsala
Uppsala, Sweden S-75123 and
Division of Physical Chemistry
Royal Institute of Technology
S-10044 Stockholm, Sweden

G. P. Littarru
Institute of Biological Chemistry
Università Cattolica S. Cuore
00168 Rome, Italy

Arne Lundin
LKB-Produkter AB
S-161 25 Bromma, Sweden

D. Maas
Medizinische Klinik
Freiburg, Federal Republic of Germany

F. E. Maly
Max-Planck-Institut für Immunbiologie
Freiburg, Federal Republic of Germany

G. Martinazzo
Laboratory Research Biodata
Rome, Italy

F. McCapra
School of Molecular Sciences
Sussex University
Palmer
Sussex, United Kingdom

G. Messeri
Clinical Chemistry Laboratory
Careggi
Florence, Italy

Gerhard Michal
Boehringer Mannheim GmbH
Research Center Tutzing
D-8132 Tutzing, Federal Republic of Germany

G. Moneti
Mass Spectrometry Unit
University of Florence
Florence, Italy

S. Müller
Robert Koch-Institut des
*   Bundesgesundheitsamtes*
Nordufer 20
D-1000 Berlin 65, West Germany

P. Neri
ISVT Sclavo
Research Center
53100 Siena, Italy

T. Olsson
Department of Clinical Chemistry
Karolinska Institute
Huddinge Hospital
S-141 86 Huddinge, Sweden

C. Orlando
Endocrinology Unit
University of Florence
Viale Morgagni 85
50134 Florence, Italy

A. Patel
Department of Medical Biochemistry
Welsh National School of Medicine
Heath Park
Cardiff CP4 4XN, United Kingdom

M. Pazzagli
Endocrinology Unit
University of Florence
Florence, Italy

B. Peskar
Pharmakologisches Institut der Universität
Freiburg, Federal Republic of Germany

A. Richardson
School of Molecular Sciences
Sussex University
Palmer
Sussex, United Kingdom

E. Th. Rietschel
Forschungsinstitut Borstel
Borstel, Federal Republic of Germany

M. Rühl
Robert Koch-Institut des
Bundesgesundheitsamtes
Nordufer 20
D-1000 Berlin 65, West Germany

M. E. T. Ryall
Department of Medical Biochemistry
Welsh National School of Medicine
Cardiff, United Kingdom

R. Salerno
Endocrinology Unit
University of Florence
Florence, Italy

K. Scheider
Robert Koch-Institut des
Bundesgesundheitsamtes
Nordufer 20
D-1000 Berlin 65, West Germany

Stanley Scher
School of Environmental Studies
Sonoma State University
Rohnert Park, California 94928

R. Scherer
Boehringer Mannheim GmbH
Research Center Tutzing
8132 Tutzing, Federal Republic of Germany

B. Schiessl
Immunogenetics Laboratory
Kinderpoliklinik der Universität
8000 Munich, Federal Republic of Germany

S. Scholz
Immunogenetics Laboratory
Kinderpoliklinik der Universität
8000 Munich, Federal Republic of Germany

E. Schram
Institute of Molecular Biology
Vrije Universiteit Brussel
Brussels, Belgium

F. Schröder
Klinisches Institut für Herzinfarktforschung
Medizinishe Universitätsklinik
Bergheimer Strasse 58
D-6900 Heidelberg, West Germany

Hartmut R. Schroeder
Ames Research and Development Laboratory
Miles Laboratories, Inc.
P.O. Box 70
Elkhart, Indiana 46515

M. Serio
Endocrinology Unit
University of Florence
Viale Morgagni 85
50134 Florence, Italy and
Chair of Endocrinology
University of Sassari
Sassari, Italy

B. Simon
Klinisches Institut für Herzinfarktforschung
Medizinische Universitätsklinik
Bergheimer Strasse 58
D-6900 Heidelberg, West Germany

D. Sławinska
Institute of Physics and Chemistry
Agricultural University
60–637 Poznań, Poland

J. Sławinski
Institute of Physics and Chemistry
Agricultural University
60–637 Poznań, Poland

F. Stähler
Boehringer Mannheim GmbH
Research Center Tutzing
P.O. Box 120
8132 Tutzing, Federal Republic of Germany

Hj. Staudinger
Max-Planck-Institut für Immunbiologie
Freiburg, Federal Republic of Germany

P. Tarli
ISVT Sclavo
Research Center
53100 Siena, Italy

U. Thalmann
Städtisches Krankenhaus Heckeshorn
Am Grossen Wannsee 80
D-1000 Berlin 39, West Germany

A. Thore
Department of Clinical Chemistry
Karolinska Institute
Huddinge Hospital
S-141 86 Huddinge, Sweden

A. Tommasi
Endocrinology Unit
University of Florence
Florence, Italy

Ch. Treffert
Boehringer Mannheim GmbH
Research Center Tutzing
8132 Tutzing, Federal Republic of Germany

Shimon Ulitzer
Department of Food Engineering and
*   Biotechnology*
Technion
Haifa 32000, Israel

L. Vermeulen
Department of Internal Medicine
State University of Ghent
Academisch Ziekenhuis
De Pintelaan 135
B-9000 Ghent, Belgium

J. Wannlund
Chemistry Department
University of California
La Jolla, California 92093

Richard A. Wecher
Department of Biology
Sonoma State University
Rohnert Park, California 94928

I. Weeks
Department of Medical Biochemistry
Welsh National School of Medicine
Cardiff, United Kingdom

H. Wokalek
Universitätshautklinik
Freiburg, Federal Republic of Germany

J. S. Woodhead
Department of Medical Biochemistry
Welsh National School of Medicine
Heath Park
Cardiff CP4 4XN, United Kingdom

Karl Wulff
Boehringer Mannheim GmbH
Research Center Tutzing
P.O. Box 120
8132 Tutzing, Federal Republic of Germany

Luminescent Assays: Perspectives in Endocrinology and Clinical Chemistry, edited by
M. Serio and M. Pazzagli, Raven Press,
New York © 1982.

Fundamental Aspects of Bioluminescent Reactions Used in Clinical Chemistry

E. Schram

Institute of Molecular Biology, Vrije Universiteit Brussel, Brussels, Belgium

It is the purpose of the present paper to summarize some general aspects of bioluminescence, more particularly those most relevant to the applications that will be discussed in the following papers. More information on the fundamental aspects is to be found in various reviews and monographs (2, 3, 10, 13, 14, 15, 16).

First of all we wish to remind the reader not quite familiar with the topic, of a few historical data about the development of our present knowledge. Although bioluminescence has been observed since antiquity its study started actually with the work of Dubois as indicated in the survey below. During a first period lasting until ca. 1950 bioluminescence has been studied from the point of view of classical biology. The introduction of more sophisticated instruments and methods after this initial period led to new developments and to our present knowledge of the molecular aspects of bioluminescence as well as to its use as an analytical tool.

Historical survey of bioluminescence:

1885   Dubois: introduction of the "luciferin" and "luciferase" concepts.

1913   Harvey: first publication on bioluminescence followed by several monographs until his death in 1959.
    1920: "The Nature of Animal Light"
    1952: "Bioluminescence"
    1957: "A History of Bioluminescence"

1947   McElroy (18): role of ATP in firefly bioluminescence

1952   Strehler and Totter (23): use of firefly luciferase for analytical purposes

1953   Strehler (24): role of NADH in bacterial bioluminescence

1956   Green and McElroy (9) : crystallization of firefly luciferase

1957   Bitler and McElroy (1) : crystallization of firefly luciferin

1960   Shimomura et al.: calcium-triggered photoproteins (Aequora, Renilla)

1961   White et al. (25): synthesis of firefly luciferin

    Cormier, DeLuca, Hastings, McCapra, et al.: biochemical and biophysical study of bioluminescence (reaction mechanisms, structure of emitting substances, quantum efficiency, etc.)

Now   Analytical applications of bioluminescence.

1

Bioluminescence is a widespread phenomenon in Nature and occurs among a great variety of organisms not even related to each other and many of which have not yet been studied extensively. A general feature of bioluminescence is that the generation of light requires rather high amounts of energy (50-60 Kcal per Einstein in the visible range) which must be accumulated in the emitting molecular species. This is apparently the reason why bioluminescence proceeds from oxidation reactions. The reactions encountered in bioluminescent systems and of interest for analytical purposes belong to the following types:

OXIDASES: $O_2 \to H$

$$XH + O_2 \to X + O_2^- + H^+$$

Ex. xanthine oxidase, NADPH oxidase (phagocytosis)

$$XH_2 + O_2 \to X + H_2O_2$$

Ex. uricase, glucose oxidase, etc.

OXYGENASES: $O_2 \to S$

a) Dioxygenases:

intramolecular: $X + O_2 \to XO_2$

Ex. firefly luciferase

intermolecular: $X_1 + X_2 + O_2 \to X_1O + X_2O$

b) Monooxygenases (mixed function oxidases)

external: $O_2 + X + AH_2 \to XO + A + H_2O$

Ex. bacterial luciferase

internal: $O_2 + XH_2 \to XO + H_2O$

PEROXIDASES: $S + H_2O_2 \to SO + H_2O$

Ex. Diplocardia longa

Horseradish

Myeloperoxidase

Microperoxidase

Superoxide ions are responsible for a faint spontaneous luminescence; the latter can be amplified by addition of oxidizable luminescent substrates, such as luminol, oxalate esters or acridine salts. The same substances can be used to produce luminescence in the presence of the H_2O_2 produced by oxidases. This luminescence should be considered as aspecific, compared with that produced by the firefly, bacterial and Diplocardia longa systems.

Hydrogen peroxide may act on biological substrates (Diplocardia luciferin) or synthetic substances; in the same way the catalyst may be inorganic (potassium ferricyanide) or biological (peroxidases). From the foregoing it must therefore be clear that it is not always easy to draw a borderline between "chemi"- and "bio"-luminescent reactions. The same remark holds for the mechanisms by which organic and biological substrates are oxidized. Mechanistic studies have indeed shown that the oxidation of both firefly luciferin and oxalate esters proceed through the formation of an intermediate dioxetane ring.

The luciferin substrates encountered in bioluminescent organisms belong to a few types that can be classified as follows:

1. THIAZOL (firefly)

2. ALDEHYDE

   a) luminescent bacteria

   $$CH_3-(CH_2)_n-C\begin{smallmatrix}O\\H\end{smallmatrix} \xrightarrow{O_2} R-C\begin{smallmatrix}O\\OH\end{smallmatrix}$$

   b) Diplocardia longa (earthworm)

   $$\xrightarrow{H_2O_2} R-C\begin{smallmatrix}O\\OH\end{smallmatrix}$$

   c) Latia (mollusc)

   (enol formate)

3. PYRAZINE

   a) Cypridina (arthropod)
   b) Renilla, Aequora (coelenterates)

It can be concluded from this survey that luciferins of a similar type may occur in organisms with no philogenetic or evolutionary relationship. A novel light emitting compound involving a polypyrrole structure has recently been identified by Dunlap et al. (5).

Although bacterial luminescence was used by Harvey in 1928 (11) for the measurement of O_2, and the analytical uses of firefly luciferase were developed by Strehler and Totter as soon as 1952 (23), the actual development of bioluminescence for analytical purposes started but 10-15 years ago. A kind of breakthrough occurred around 1978 when a choice of specific instruments were made available and purified reagents put on the market by several manufacturers. Thanks to these improvements the applications of bioluminescence could be developed in various directions, and still new developments may be anticipated soon. The following table gives a short survey of the systems presently used. Additional information can be found in the proceedings of two symposia held respectively in Brussels (21) and San Diego (4). The clinical applications are dealt with in two survey papers (8 ,26) as well as in a monograph to be published shortly (17).

Analytical applications of bioluminescent systems:

System	Substrates	Applications
Firefly	Luciferin ATP	Biomass (bacteriuria, antibiograms, etc.) Enzymes (kinases) and their substrates
Bacteria	Aldehyde $FMNH_2$ $NAD(P)H$	Enzymes (dehydrogenases) and their substrates
Peroxidases HRP Microperoxidase Diplocardia	H_2O_2 + luminol or luciferin	Enzymes (oxidases) and their substrates Luminescent tags (immunoassays)
Photoproteins	Luciferin	Ca^{++}

When dealing with the applications of luminescent reactions one should remember that, contrary to other methods, the assays are based on the measurement of a reaction velocity. The kinetics of the reaction is therefore of paramount importance besides, of course, more trivial factors as quantum efficiency, emission spectrum, temperature, etc. This particular aspects are discussed here in more detail for the two best studied bioluminescent systems.

Bacterial luciferase.

According to the work of Hastings and his group (14,15) the reaction scheme may be summarized as follows:

$$NAD^+ \quad FMNH_2 + E \rightleftharpoons E\text{-}FH_2 \xrightarrow{O_2} E\text{-}FH \xrightarrow{RCHO} E\text{-}FH$$

$$NADH \quad FMN + H_2O_2$$

$$E + FMN + H_2O_2$$

(E = Enzyme)

Reduced FMN is very unstable and oxidizes spontaneously in less than a second with the production of H_2O_2 unless it is bound by the enzyme. Although the enzyme is able to turn over it will therefore react only once when one starts from preformed $FMNH_2$. In most cases the latter will be produced extemporaneously from $NAD(P)H$ in the presence of FMN reductase which is found associated with the luciferase in luminescent bacteria. Two reductases have been isolated (7), specific for NAD or NADP, which makes it possible to assay these nucleotides separately in the presence of added FMN.

Depending on the experimental conditions different shapes can be obtained for the luminescence time curve. When starting from preformed

NAD(P)H the initial peak is followed by a decay whose rate will depend on the FMN reductase concentration. On the contrary, when the pyridine nucleotide is reduced in situ by a coupled reaction the curve will show an easily measurable ascending part followed by a flattened peak or a plateau. For practical purposes it is therefore important that the several enzymes (dehydrogenase, FMN reductase and luciferase) be used in the appropriate concentration ratios.

In the absence of aldehyde the complex between $FMNH_2$ and O_2 decays to FMN and H_2O_2 with a half-life of ca. 20 sec. at room temperature. It could however be isolated by Hastings and Balny (12) by chromatography at $-20°C$. The length of the aldehyde influences the half-life of the luminescent reaction but not its quantum efficiency. Discussion is still going on about the structure of the emitting molecular species which has so far not been identified with certainty. Moreover, in some bacterial strains, sensitized luminescence may occur as shown by Gast and Lee (6).

As will appear from the paper presented by Ulitzur at this symposium live luminescent bacteria can be used for various purposes, further extending the potentialities offered by the in vitro system.

Firefly luciferase.

This is by far the most popular system and an impressive amount of work has been devoted to the study of its mechanism during the last thirty years, chiefly by McElroy's group. A survey of our present knowledge in this respect was published some years ago by DeLuca (2). According to this author the mechanism of the firefly luciferase reaction may be represented in the following way:

$$LH_2 + ATP\text{-}Mg + \bigcirc \underset{1}{\rightleftharpoons} \overset{LH_2}{\underset{}{\bigcirc}}\text{-}ATP \underset{2}{\rightleftharpoons} \bigcirc\text{-}LH_2AMP$$

$$3 \updownarrow \quad \text{Proton abstraction}$$

$$\bigcirc\text{-}LHAMP$$

$$\updownarrow \quad \text{Conformational change}$$

$$AMP + CO_2 + \bigcirc\text{-}P + h\nu \xleftarrow{O_2} \square\text{-}LHAMP$$

$$LH_2 = \text{D-Luciferin}$$

$$P \quad = \text{Oxyluciferin}$$

An additional step should be added to this scheme, i.e. the release of the end-product from the enzyme. Since this process occurs rather slowly higher ATP concentrations will tend to inhibit the enzyme and a more or less rapid decrease of the luminescence will be observed. As shown by Schram et al. (22) the shape of the luminescence time-curve can be interpreted on the basis of the following two overall reactions:

$$LH_2 + ATP + O_2 + E \xrightarrow{k_1} E\text{-}LO + AMP + CO_2 + h\nu$$

$$E\text{-}LO \xrightarrow{k_2} E + LO$$

If L_0 corresponds to the initial luminescence before the occurrence of enzyme inhibition, and L_e to the steady state luminescence due to the slow turn-over of the enzyme after it has undergone inhibition, one finds that the luminescence varies with time according to the following equation (obtained by integration):

$$L_t = \frac{L_o\,(k_2 + k_1 e^{-(k_1 + k_2)t})}{k_1 + k_2}$$

This equation holds for the case where the ATP concentration is considerably higher than the enzyme concentration and can be considered constant during the experiment. (see Fig. 1)

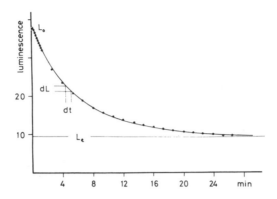

Fig. 1. Time course of luciferase light reaction (enzyme 3.85×10^{-9}M, ATP 1.16×10^{-6}M and luciferin 3.33×10^{-5}M; — computed curve, ······ experimental figures).

At low ATP concentrations and when the enzyme is rather concentrated the decrease of the luminescence must be ascribed to the consumption

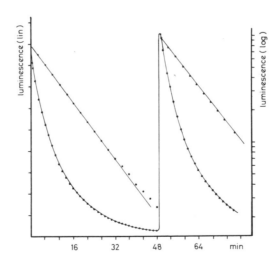

Fig. 2. Time course of luminescence upon successive additions of ATP (enzyme 4.8×10^{-8}M, luciferin 4.1×10^{-4}M, ATP 5.6×10^{-9}M right after each addition).

of the ATP rather than to the inhibition of the enzyme. In this opposite situation the luminescence decreases exponentially without appre-
ciable enzyme inhibition, as illustrated in figure 2.
In practice an intermediate situation may of course be encountered.
For analytical purposes it is however advisable to choose experimental
conditions such that ATP consumption and enzyme inhibition are reduced
to a minimum. A more or less constant steady state luminescence is then
obtained which can easily be measured. The achievement of this goal
can be facilitated by the addition of pyrophosphate (and other substances) which seemingly accelerates the release of the end-product, as visible in figure 3. Excess of pyrophosphate should be avoided in order
not to inhibit the luminescent reaction itself. The effect of pyrophosphate has been observed from the beginning (19) but was neglected
for many years until its usefulness was rediscovered.

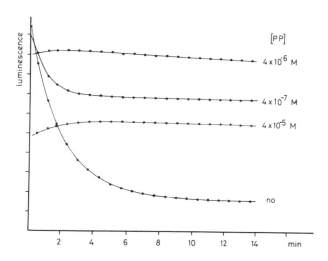

Fig. 3. Effect of pyrophosphate on the luminescence time-course (enzyme 4 x 10^{-9}M, luciferin 3 x 10^{-5}M, ATP 1.3 x 10^{-1}M).

    In conclusion it may be said that the analytical potentialities of
ATP bioluminescence seem now well established. The applications of bacterial luminescence although potentially as important as those of firefly luciferase, would certainly deserve to be developed further. A
promising system that has been studied but recently (5) deals with the
earthworm Diplocardia longa. Contrary to the preceding systems H_2O_2 is
involved in the oxidation of the luciferin substrate, instead of oxygen.
Thanks to its sensitivity and linearity over a wide dynamic range it
could evolve into a basic method for the assay of H_2O_2 produced by oxidases, now measured by luminol luminescence.
    As will appear from the other presentations at this symposium
bioluminescent reactions lend themselves to the most diversified applications; the most striking development in this respect is probably the
use of luminescent reactions for the replacement of radioactivity in
immunoassays.

REFERENCES

1. Bitler, B. and McElroy, W.D. (1957): The preparation and properties of crystalline firefly luciferin. Arch. Biochem. Biophys., 72: 358-368.

2. DeLuca, M. (1976): Firefly Luciferase. Adv. Enzymol., 44: 37-68.

3. DeLuca, M.A., editor (1978): Bioluminescence and Chemiluminescence. Meth. Enzymol., vol. 57, Acad. Press, New York.

4. DeLuca, M.A. and McElroy, W.D., editors (1981): Bioluminescence and Chemiluminescence, Acad. Press, New York.

5. Dunlap, J.C., Hastings, J.W. and Shimomura, O. (1980): Crossreactivity between the light-emitting systems of distantly related organisms: novel type of light-emitting compound. Proc. Natl. Acad. Sci. USA, 77: 1394-1397.

6. Gast, R. and Lee, J. (1978): Isolation of in vivo emitter in bacterial luminescence. Proc. Natl. Acad. Sci. USA., 75: 833-837.

7. Gerlo, E. and Charlier, J. (1975): Identification of NADH-specific and NADPH-specific FMN reductases in Beneckea harveyi. Eur. J. Biochem., 57: 461-467.

8. Gorus, F. and Schram, E. (1979): Applications of bio- and chemiluminescence in the clinical laboratory. Clin. Chem., 25: 512-519.

9. Green, A.A. and McElroy, W.D. (1956): Crystalline firefly luciferase. Biochem. Biophys. Acta, 20: 170-176.

10. Hart, R.C. and Cormier, M.J. (1979): Recent advances in the mechanisms of bio- and chemiluminescent reactions. Photochem. Photobiol., 29: 209-215.

11. Harvey, E.N. (1928), Plant Physiol., 3: 85

12. Hastings, J.W. and Balny, C. (1975): The oxygenated bacterial luciferase-flavin intermediate. J. Biol. Chem., 250: 7288-7293.

13. Hastings, J.W. and Wilson, Th. (1976): Bioluminescence and Chemiluminescence. Photochem. Photobiol., 23: 461-473.

14. Hastings, J.W. and Nealson, K.H. (1977): Bacterial Bioluminescence. Ann. Rev. Microbiol., 31: 549-595.

15. Hastings, J.W. (1978): The Chemistry and Biology of Bacterial Light Emission. Photochem. Photobiol., 27: 397-404.

16. Herring, P.J., editor (1978): Bioluminescence in Action, Acad. Press New York.

17. Kricka, L.J. and Carter, T.J.N., editors (in press): Clinical and biochemical applications of luminescence, Dekker, New York.

18. McElroy, W.D. (1947): The energy source for bioluminescence in an isolated system. Proc. Natl. Acad. Sci. USA, 33: 342-345.

19. McElroy, W.D., Hastings, J.W., Coulombre, J. and Sonnenfeld, V. (1953): The mechanism of action of pyrophosphate in firefly luminescence. Arch. Biochem. Biophys., 46: 399-416.

20. Rudie, N.G., Mulkerrin, M.G. and Wampler, J.E. (1981): Earthworm Bioluminescence: Characterization of high specific activity Diplocardia longa luciferase and the reaction it catalyzes. Biochem. 20: 344-350.

21. Schram, E. and Stanley, P.E., editors (1979): Analytical Applications of Bioluminescence and Chemiluminescence, State Printing and Publishing, Inc., Westlake Village, CA 91361.

22. Schram, E., Ahmad, M. and Moreels, E. (1981): Use of a mathematical representation for the time-course of the firefly luciferase light reaction. In: Bioluminescence and Chemiluminescence, edited by M.A. DeLuca and W.D. McElroy, pp. 491-496, Acad. Press, New York.

23. Strehler, B.L. and Totter, J.R. (1952): Firefly luminescence in the study of energy transfer mechanisms. Arch. Biochem. Biophys., 40: 28-41.

24. Strehler, B.L. (1953): Luminescence in cell-free extracts of luminous bacteria and its activation by DPN. J. Am. Chem. Soc., 75: 1264

25. White, E.H., McCapra, F., Field, G. and McElroy, W.D. (1961): The structure and synthesis of firefly luciferin. J. Am. Chem. Soc., 83: 2402-2403.

26. Whitehead, Th. P., Kricka, L.J., Carter, T.J.N. and Thorpe, G.H.G. (1979): Analytical luminescence: Its potential in the clinical laboratory. Clin. Chem., 25: 1531-1546.

Acknowledgements.
This work was supported by a grant of the Belgian Government (Programmatie van het Wetenschapsbeleid).

Luminescent Assays: Perspectives in Endocrinology and Clinical Chemistry, edited by M. Serio and M. Pazzagli, Raven Press, New York © 1982.

General Applications of Bioluminescence in the Clinical Laboratory

Larry J. Kricka

Department of Clinical Chemistry, Wolfson Research Laboratories, University of Birmingham, Birmingham B15 2TH, United Kingdom

The "clinical laboratory" is comprised of a series of loosely associated disciplines, clinical chemistry, haematology, bacteriology, virology, etc (Fig 1) responsible for the analysis of a variety of body components known to be of value in the detection, diagnosis and management of disease. Many of the analyses performed are for substances present at very low concentrations and an additional problem is that only a very limited amount of the specimen may be available (eg, paediatric specimens). Thus highly sensitive analytical methods are both desirable and necessary.

The different types of chemiluminescent and bioluminescent reactions, involving for example, luminol/peroxide, firefly luciferase/luciferin/adenosine triphosphate (ATP), (26), can be used as the basis of extremely sensitive analytical methods. The clinical laboratory has realised their potential and a number of applications have been described. Basically, chemiluminescent and bioluminescent reactions allow the highly sensitive determination of peroxide, the reduced form of nicotinamide adenine dinucleotide (NADH) and ATP. These substances are intermediates in numerous assays, particularly in clinical chemistry. When considering the introduction of a new analytical technique, such as luminescence into the laboratory, the range of applications, and availability of suitable instrumentation and reagents are key issues.

APPLICATIONS

Some representative examples of luminescent analyses taken from the various clinical laboratory disciplines are outlined in the following sections. In many cases the applications are at an early stage of development and there has been only a limited number of reports of comparisons with conventional non-luminescent methods.

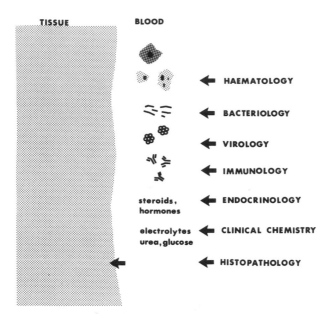

FIG 1.   Schematic representation of clinical laboratory
          analyses.

Haematology and Blood Banking

Most attention has been directed towards the measurement
of ATP levels in red blood cells and platelets. ATP levels
correlate with the viability of a red blood cell. Thus the
measurement of ATP has been advocated as a pre-transfusion
test of the viability of blood which has been stored
frozen (5). The principle of the method is shown in
Fig. 2, and involves release of ATP from cells and
subsequent quantitation using the firefly luciferase
reaction.

Bacteriology

Conventional methods for detecting bacteriuria (eg,
culture) are slow and labour intensive. Bioluminescent
assay of bacterial ATP offers a very rapid and sensitive

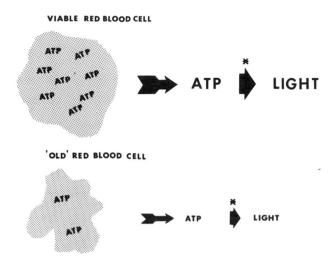

FIG 2. Application of the firefly luciferase reaction in determining viability of red blood cells (<u>via</u> ATP content).

method of detecting bacteriuria (5). Fig. 3 illustrates the principle of the assay. Non-bacterial cells present in the urine specimen are lysed and the ATP destroyed with apyrase. Bacterial ATP is then released and quantitated using the firefly luciferase reaction. The amount of ATP correlates directly with the number of cells present and the method is able to detect approximately 10^5 bacterial cells/ml, a cell count which is accepted as representing significant bacteriuria (7).

Immunology

An exciting application of luminescence is in the study of phagocytosis. Activation of a phagocytic cell, eg, a polymorphonuclear leukocyte (PMN), by a phagocytosable particle is accompanied by a burst of chemiluminescence which may be amplified by luminol. The chemiluminescence arises as a result of reactions involving superoxide anions, hydroxyl radicals and hydrogen peroxide. The phagocytic process involves a preliminary activation (opsonization) by a group of serum proteins known as "opsonins" which promote

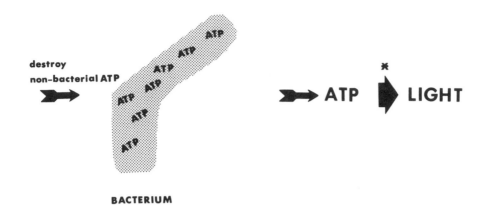

FIG 3. Application of firefly luciferase reaction to
        determine the presence of bacteria (<u>via</u> ATP
        content).

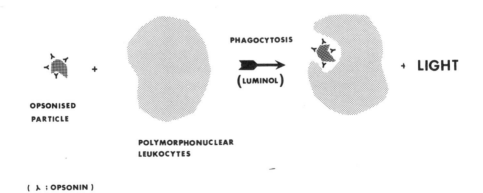

FIG 4. Schematic representation of the phagocytic
        process. (Luminol enhances the burst of
        luminescence which accompanies phagocytosis).

the binding of a particle to a PMN prior to its engulfment and destruction (Fig. 4). Luminescence has been used to study the patency of both the activation processes and the processes within the PMN.

Preliminary results indicate that luminescent assays may prove to be a valuable tool in detecting and assessing immune competence in a variety of disorders, eg, chronic granulomatous disease of childhood (21).

Clinical Chemistry

Luminescent assays for a large number of the substances routinely measured by the clinical chemistry laboratory have been reported (26) (Table 1). In most cases the principle of the assay is unchanged and a luminescent indicator reaction merely replaces a conventional colorimetric or spectrophotometric reaction. Three typical examples, luminescent assays for cholesterol, alcohol and creatine kinase, are illustrated in Fig. 5.

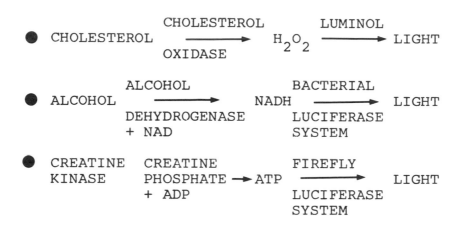

FIG. 5. Principles of the luminescent assays of cholesterol, alcohol and creatine kinase.

The sensitivity of luminescent reactions has prompted the investigation of luminescence as an alternative to radioactivity in immunoassay. Several different types of luminescent immunoassay have been explored involving luminescent labels, eg, luminol (16), firefly luciferase (24), luminescent detection of co-factors, eg, ATP (3) NADH (15), and luminescent detection of conventional labels, eg, horseradish peroxidase (23). Detection limits

TABLE 2

Commercially available luminometers[a]

Model	Company
Automated Luminescence Analyser	Alpkem Corp
Chem-Glow Photometer	American Instrument Company
Autolight 101, Monolight 201, 301, 401	Analytical Luminescence Lab Inc
Biolumat LB9500	Berthhold Laboratorium
Biometer 760	Du Pont
Photometre Pico-ATP	Jobin Yvon SA
Luminometer 1250	LKB Wallac
Celltester, Lumacounter, Biocounter: 1010, 1030, 1060, 1070, 2000, 2010, 2080	Lumac
Luminescence Analyser, 302, 340/50	Marwell International, AB
Lumitran 2000	New Brunswick Scientific Co Inc
Pico-Lite 6100	Packard Instrument Co Inc
ATP Photometer 100, 2000, 3000	SAI Technology Inc
Bioluminescence Analyzer XP-2000-2	Skan AG
ATP Photometer 20	Turner Designs
Surface Reaction Photometer II, IIs, III	Vitatect Corp

[a] More extensive details are to be found in Stanley, P.E. (1981). Instrumentation In: Clinical and Biochemical Applications of Luminescence, edited by L.J. Kricka and T.J.N. Carter, in press, Marcel Dekker, New York.

circulation of a cooling fluid, eg, LKB Luminometer, whilst others allow selection of a temperature within a specific range, eg, Pico-Lite (5-44°C).

Portable

Luminescence has some applications which are "extra-laboratory" and these require a portable luminometer, and several portable machines are now available, eg, SAI ATP Photometer Model 100.

REAGENTS

Currently the number of luminescent reagents available is limited. Several manufacturers sell the chemiluminescent compounds luminol and lucigenin specially purified for luminescent work. However, these are not the most efficient chemiluminescent compounds known. Some annelated analogues of luminol are up to 300% more efficient than luminol (11), and it is anticipated that compounds like this will eventually be available commercially.

Reagents for the bioluminescent firefly and marine bacterial reactions are available in purified form from several companies (LKB, Analytical Luminescence Laboratories, Boehringer Corporation) and a comparison of the relative performance of the different firefly reagents has been published (25). The phenomenon of bioluminescence occurs widely, and an exciting prospect for the future will be the identification of further bioluminescent reactions of value in clinical laboratory analyses.

REFERENCES

1.   Arakawa, H., Maeda, M. and Tsuki, A. (1977) : Bunseki Kagaku, 26 : 322-326.

2.   Brolin, S.E., Wettermark, G. and Hammer, H. (1977) : Strahlentherapie, 153 : 124-131.

3.   Carrico, J.R., Yeung, K.K., Schroeder, H.R., Boguslaski, R.C., Buckler, R.T. and Christner, J.E. (1976) : Anal. Biochem., 76 : 95-110.

4.   Haggerty, C., Jablonski, E., Stav, L. and De Luca, M. (1978) : Anal. Biochem., 88 : 162-173.

5.   Harber, M.J. (1981) : In: Clinical and Biochemical Applications of Luminescence, edited by L.J. Kricka and T.J.N. Carter, in press. Marcel Dekker, New York.

6.   Hercules, D.M. and Sheehan, T.L. (1978) : Anal. Chem., 50 : 20-25.

7.   Kass, E.H. (1957) : Arch. Intern. Med., 100 : 709-714.

8.   Kricka, L.J. and Carter, T.J.N. (1981) : In: <u>Clinical and Biochemical Applications of Luminescence</u>, edited by L.J. Kricka and T.J.N. Carter, in press. Marcel Dekker New York.

9.   Lundin, A., Rickardsson, A. and Thore, A. (1976) : <u>Anal. Biochem.</u>, 75 : 611-620.

10. Maier, C. (1977) : <u>Belgian Patent</u> 856,182.

11. McCapra, F. (1966) : <u>Q. Rev. (Lond).</u>, 20: 485-510.

12. Neufeld, H.A., Conklin, C.J. and Towner, R.D. (1965): <u>Anal. Biochem.</u>, 12: 303-309.

13. Nicholas, D.J.D. and Clarke, G.R. (1971) : <u>Anal. Biochem.</u>, 42: 560-568.

14. Njus, D., Baldwin, T.O. and Hastings, J.W. (1974): <u>Anal. Biochem.</u>, 61: 280-287.

15. Schroeder, H.R., Carrico, R.J., Boguslaski, R.C. and Christner, J.E. (1976): <u>Anal. Biochem.</u>, 72: 283-292.

16. Schroeder, H.R., Vogelhut, P.O., Carrico, R.J., Boguslaski, R.C. and Buckler, R.T. (1976) : <u>Anal. Chem.</u> 48: 1933-1937.

17. Schroeder, H.R., Yeager, F.M., Boguslaski, R.C., Snoke, E.O. and Buckler, E.T. (1977) : <u>Clin. Chem.</u>, 23: 1132. Abstract.

18. Sheehan, T.L. and Hercules, D.M. (1977) : <u>Anal. Chem.</u>, 49: 446-450.

19. Stanley, P.E. (1974) : In: <u>Liquid Scintillation Counting</u>, edited by M.A. Crook and P. Johnson pp 253-271, Heyden, London.

20. Strehler, B.L. (1968) : <u>Methods Biochem. Anal.</u>, 16: 99-181.

21. Trush, M.A., Wilson, M.E. and Van Dyker, K. (1978) : <u>Methods Enzymol.</u>, 57: 462-494.

22. Ulitzur, S. and Hastings, J.W. (1978): <u>Proc. Natl. Acad. Sci. USA</u>, 75: 266-269.

23. Velan, B. and Halmann, M. (1978) : <u>Immunochemistry</u>, 15: 331-333.

24. Wannlund, J., Azari, J., Levine, L. and DeLuca, M. (1980): <u>Biochem. Biophys. Res. Commun.</u>, 96: 440-446.

25. Webster, J.J., Chang, J.C., Howard, J.L. and Leach, F.R. (1979): <u>J. Appl. Biochem.</u> 1: 471-478.

26. Whitehead, T.P., Kricka, L.J., Carter, T.J.N. and Thorpe, G.H.G. (1979): <u>Clin. Chem.</u>, 25: 1531-1546.

Luminescent Assays: Perspectives in Endocrinology and Clinical Chemistry, edited by M. Serio and M. Pazzagli, Raven Press, New York © 1982.

Automatic Instrumentation for Chemi- and Bioluminescence Assays

Fritz Berthold and Helmut Kubisiak

Laboratorium Prof. Dr. Berthold, D-7547 Wildbad, Federal Republic of Germany

After having gained several years of experience with manual luminescence analyzers we were faced with an increasing demand for automation.

A great problem for the instrument designer is that as yet there is no generally accepted routine application of either bio- or chemiluminescence (CL). At this stage, therefore, automatic instruments should be as flexible as possible. In particular, we looked at three areas of luminescence applications: phagocytosis or cell stimulation, microbiology and luminescence immuno-assay (LIA).

In order to assay phagocytosis and cell stimulation one usually observes the time dependent CL rate over a period of, say, 5-100 minutes. Very high sensitivity is desired, requiring a photon counter, possibly with cooled cathode. Temperature stabilisation is necessary. The number of samples is typically well below 20.

In microbiology the situation is different. Counting times are only around 10 - 20 s, sample numbers between 20 and 500 might be typical. Reagent injection (e.g. luciferin/luciferase) is required, high sensitivity is also needed.

In LIA the sample capacity should be between 100 and 1000 samples for a clinical instrument. Counting times are typically 10 s, an automatic injector (for corrosive reagents) is required.

Thanks to our close cooperation with the Freiburg Research Group around H. Fischer, our first automatic luminescence analyzer was primarily oriented towards the assay of CL associated with phagocytosis and cell stimulation. A first report was given on the San Diego Conference 1980 (1), and I will only point out the progress made since then.

The instrument (FIG. 1) measures six samples simultaneously using six photomultiplier (pm) tubes and detector assemblies. Since it is not possible to get identical sensitivities for six pm-tubes each tube is calibrated once with a standard light source and the results are normalized automatically by the microcomputer. This standardization is provided for four different wave lengths so that 24 sensitivity constants can be stored and applied.

Temperatures are preset by keyboard, actual as well as preset temperature values are displayed. Each channel is started independently. Count rates and integrated counts can be printed out in time intervals from 0,6 s to beyond 60 minutes.

The best presentation and evaluation of data is obtained by means of a computer directly connected with the instrument, so that histograms may be visualized on a video screen.

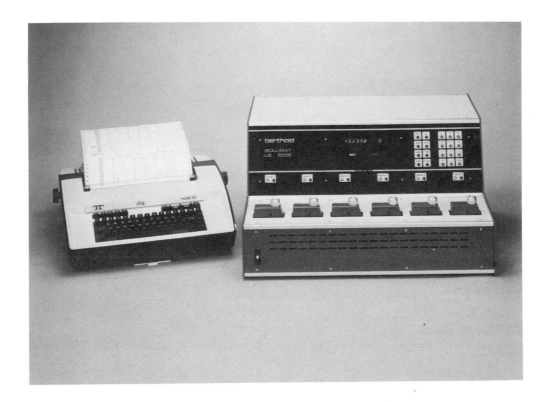

FIG. 1: Six-channel Luminescence Analyzer with six detectors for simul-
        taneous assay, microprocessor version

     The demands with regard to automation are different when we leave
phagocytosis and consider microbiology or LIA. In the latter areas a
sample is measured only once during a short time (< 30 s). Furthermore,
the sample number is much larger, so that sequential instead of parallel
measurement is indicated.
     Our first decision was to use discrete sample analysis and not flow
analysis. This decision was practically forced upon us when considering
solid-phase LIA's and other applications where carrier fluids are
excluded.
     Schroeder et al. (2) described a remarkable instrument for LIA's
carried out in a multiwell plastic plate. In spite of certain obvious
advantages in using microtiter plates we chose discrete vials 12 mm diameter, 35 - 55 mm high.
     Our reasons were
1. most favorable geometry of the vials directly in front of the pm-tube,
   leading to higher sensitivity

2. perfect optical separation of the sample actually measured with regard to all others
3. high flexibility of sample formate. The vial might contain the sample directly or it might serve as an auxiliary container for microtiter cups or coated spheres.

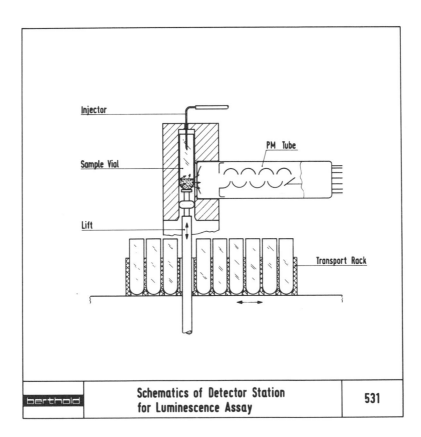

FIG. 2: Schematics of Detector Station for Luminescence Assay

    The individual vials are placed into racks and moved to the detector station (FIG. 2). In the measuring position, the sample is lifted into a light-tight measuring chamber in front of the pm-tube. If reagent addition is required, an automatic injector adds a preset volume of 50 - 500 μl of reagent to the sample. We have also foreseen active mixing of the reagents with the sample if necessary.
    Based on this design we developed two instruments primarily distinguished by their sample capacity.

FIG. 3 shows the concept of a thousand-sample luminescence analyzer.

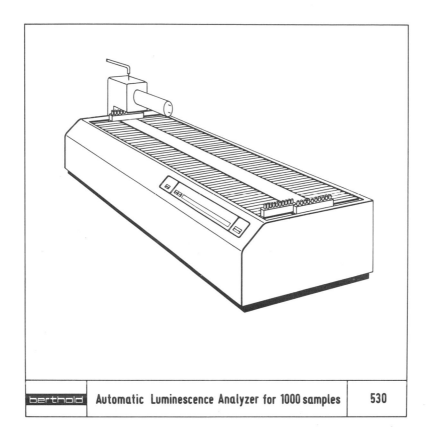

Automatic Luminescence Analyzer for 1000 samples   530

FIG. 3: Automatic Luminescence Analyzer for 1000 samples

100 racks carry up to 10 vials each. The arrangement and transport of racks follows the principle of the horizontal paternoster frequently applied for fraction collectors or automatic gamma counters. This instrument should be useful for LIA's in clinical scale, in clinical or industrial application of microbiology, as well as other areas.

Before finalizing the thousand-sample analyzer, we built an instrument for 20 samples only (FIG. 4). One single rack carries 20 vials in a linear motion to the detector station already described.

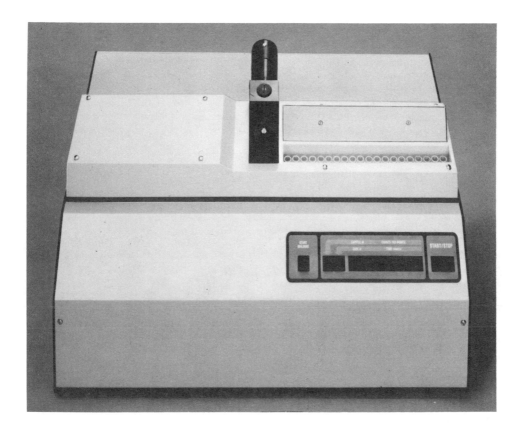

FIG. 4: Automatic Luminescence Analyzer for 20 samples

This instrument has two additional features:
1. samples may be measured repetitively. After having measured each sample once, the rack returns to its initial position and repeats the process
2. samples (and detector assembly) can be temperature stabilized, with precise adjustion in steps of 0,1°C between 25 and 50°C.

While the thousand-sample instrument mentioned before is clearly aimed at clinical or industrial applications, the 20 channel analyzer addresses the field between research and routine applications, which is perhaps characteristic for the present situation in bio- and chemiluminescence. Examples might be antibiograms, general microbial analyses, immunoassay, or phagocytosis with slow cinetics where simultaneous counting with the six-channel instrument may not be required.

All instruments described are microprocessor-controlled and have the option of (a) direct print-out of data on teletype lister printer or (b) direct connection to computers via a V-24 interface.

A final word on some key components. For high sensitivity photon detection, there is no practical alternative to pm-tubes. We operate pm-tubes in the photon counting mode because this is the only way to

obtain high sensitivity as well as stability (3). However, the requirements for photomultiplier quality as well as for fast and sensitive
electronics are higher in photon counting than for d.c. operation.

Another function which has to be designed with great care is reagent
injection. It is, unfortunately, not trivial to design injectors for
reagent volumes variable from 50 to 500 µl, sometimes with required
precisions better than 1 %, for strongly corrosive liquids which should
not damage the injection system, which should never lose one drop when
not actuated, and never ejecting if no vial is in position. Remember that
this is a problem not existing in radio-immunoassay since nuclear radia-
tion is emitted spontaneously without a chemical activator (of course I
realize that just this fact also relates to the potentially higher sensitivity of LIA with regard to RIA).

REFERENCES:

1. Berthold, F., Ernst, M., Fischer, H., and Kubisiak, H. (1981): Six-
   channel luminescence analyzer for phagocytosis applications. In:
   Bioluminescence and Chemiluminescence, ed. by DeLuca, M.A., and
   McElroy, W.D., pp. 699-703.
2. Schroeder, H.R., Hines, C.M., and Vogelhut, P.O. (1981): Chemiluminescence Immunoassay for anti-human IgG. In: Bioluminescence and
   Chemiluminescence, ed. by DeLuca, M.A., and McElroy, W.D., pp. 55-61.
3. Zatzick, M.R. (1972): How to make every photon count. Electro-optical
   Systems Design, pp. 20-27.

Luminescent Assays: Perspectives in Endocrinology and Clinical Chemistry, edited by M. Serio and M. Pazzagli, Raven Press, New York © 1982.

Applications of Firefly Luciferase

Arne Lundin

LKB-Produkter AB, S-161 25 Bromma, Sweden

The firefly reaction has been used for analytical purposes since 1947 when McElroy discovered that ATP was one of the subtrates participating in this reaction (23). It was soon realized that the firefly reaction could be used for assays of all metabolites and enzymes participating in ATP converting reactions (29). Recently the firefly reaction has also been used for immunoanalyses (5, 28, 33, 34). Thus almost any biological compound can at least potentially be assayed either by coupled enzymatic reactions or by luminescent immunoassays using the firefly reaction as the last step in the assay.

Although several clinical applications have been suggested, firefly luminescence has not yet become a routine technique in clinical laboratories. Until recently the major obstacle for a widespread use of firefly luminescence has been the lack of highly purified and standardized firefly reagents with suitable kinetic properties. The major intention of the present paper is to show how this problem has been solved. In addition a few guidelines how to use such reagents in various analytical situations are proposed. Detailed lists on applications of firefly luminescence have been published elsewhere (14, 15) and there are several excellent reviews on clinical applications of luminescence (9, 31, 35). Thus references to specific applications will be made only to papers of general methodological interest.

THE FIREFLY LUCIFERASE REACTION

Firefly luciferases with similar but not identical structures can be isolated from several species of fireflies. Most of the scientific work has been done using the American firefly Photinus pyralis. Highly purified preparations of luciferase can be obtained from crude homogenates of firefly lanterns be several methods: 1) batch adsorption to calcium phosphate gel followed by fractionation with ammonium sulphate (10), 2) ion-exchange chromatography (2, 27), 3) affinity chromatography (4), 4) fractionation with ammonium sulphate followed by isoeletric focusing (12, 18). The fact that firefly luciferase is an euglobulin with a low solubility at low ionic strength is utilized in all four methods. After concentrating the

29

partially purified luciferase by ammonium sulphate precipitation or ultrafiltration, luciferase can be repeatedly crystallized by dialysis against a solution of low ionic strength. In method number 4 luciferase precipitates in the electrofocusing column at its isoelectric point and can be collected by centrifugation and subsequently washed with distilled water. The luciferase preparation obtained with this method is homogeneous as judged by SDS gel electrophoresis and analytical isoelectrofocusing and levels of important contaminating enzymes as e.g. adenylate kinase are low (18).

The properties of firefly luciferase have been described in detail in several reviews (6, 24). Firefly luciferase has a molecular weight of approx. 100 000 and consists of two similar subunits. It is an extremely hydrophobic protein and contains 6-7 SH groups, two of which are at the active site. There are two binding sites for luciferin and ATP per 100 000 molecular weight of enzyme. However, for the enzymatically active substrate, the Mg-ATP complex, and the substrate analog dehydroluciferyl adenylate there is only one site. The peak emission for firefly bioluminescence at optimum pH (pH 7.75) is 560 nm. At pH<7 or in the presence of Hg^{2+}, Zn^{2+} and Cd^{2+} cations a shift to red light with a peak emission at 616 nm is observed.

The structures of the substrate D-luciferin, the product oxyluciferin and the substrate analogs L-luciferin and dehydroluciferin are shown in Fig. 1. Methods for synthesis of these compounds have been described (3).

The reactions catalyzed by firefly luciferase (E) are also shown in Fig. 1. In the inital reaction, there is an adenyl group transfer from ATP to the carboxyl group of luciferin (LH_2) with the elimination of inorganic pyrophosphate (PP_i). The reaction is rapid and reversible and moderate concentrations of pyrophosphate inhibits the forward reaction.

In the second reaction the enzyme bound luciferyl adenylate (LH_2-AMP) reacts with molecular oxygen to form oxyluciferin (oxyL) in an electronically excited state, CO_2 and AMP. In this reaction two rate limiting steps (a proton abstraction from luciferin and a conformational change of luciferase) must take place before oxidation. These steps result in a 25 msec lag before any light is emitted and a 300 msec rise time before peak light emission is attained (7).

In the third reaction oxyluciferin goes from excited to ground state with emission of a photon. Under optimal conditions the quantum yield is close to unity and the emitted light is yellow-green.

In the fourth reaction oxyluciferin and AMP are released from the enzyme product complex (E·oxyL·AMP). This reaction is slow and at high substrate concentrations it leads to a consumption of the enzyme resulting in a rapid decay of the light emission.

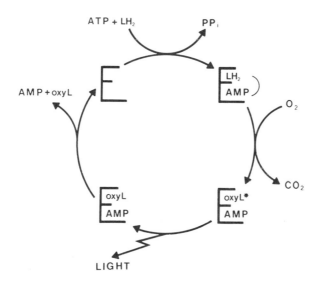

FIG. 1: Chemistry of the firefly luciferase reaction. In the upper
part of the figure the structures of the substrate D-luciferin
(LH$_2$), the product oxyluciferin (oxyL) and the substrate analogs
L-luciferin and dehydroluciferin are shown. The lower part of the
figure shows the reactions catalyzed by firefly luciferase (E). The
substrate analogs can substitute for D-luciferin in the first reaction
of the cycle, i.e. the activation of the carboxyl group, but no
further reaction to give light takes place.

KINETICS OF THE LIGHT EMISSION

The kinetics of the light emission are extremely important from an analytical point of view. When using the firefly system for monitoring of ATP converting reactions the kinetics of rise and decay of the emission will determine the time resolution and the time during which measurements can be performed. The kinetics of the rise of the emission is determined by reactions within the enzyme substrate complex ($E \cdot LH_2$-AMP) and will not be affected by changes in substrate or enzyme concentrations (7). The kinetics of the decay of the light emission, on the other hand, is strongly influenced by reaction conditions. A stable light emission, i.e. a decay <1 % /min, can only be obtained if the following requirements are fulfilled:

1) Constant ATP concentration (no ATP converting enzymes contaminating the reagent and a low (<1%/min) rate of ATP consumption in the luciferase reaction).

2) Constant luciferin concentration (preferably saturating to avoid changes of the light emission resulting from minor pipetting errors or from reactions degrading or binding luciferin).

3) Constant concentration of free luciferase (i.e. the proportion of luciferase becoming inactivated as e.g. enzyme product complex should be negligible).

4) Constant and suitable reaction conditions (constant temperature below or around $25^{\circ}C$, the temperature optimum of the reaction, constant pH in the interval 6-8 using e.g. tris acetate or imidazole acetate buffer).

With highly purified luciferase a stable light emission at low substrate concentrations is easily obtained. At high substrate concentrations the light decays mainly due to formation of enzyme product complex. However, a stable light is of analytical importance only up to the upper limit of the linear range of the firefly assay of ATP. This limit is somewhat influenced by reaction conditions and can be calculated from the K_m value for ATP using the Michaelis-Menten equation. Since the K_m value under optimal reaction conditions is 0.25 mM ATP (12) the upper limit of the linear range is approx. 1.0 µM.

The decay of the light emission obtained with 1.0 µM ATP and 0.4 mM D-luciferin is shown in Fig. 2a. The addition of a non-inhibitory concentration of PP_i (1.0 µM) results in a less rapid decay (Fig. 2b) most likely due to a destabilization of the enzyme product complex. In Fig. 2c the luciferase concentration is approx. 2 fold higher while the luciferase activity is kept at the same level as in Fig. 2a-b by addition of the competitive inhibitor L-luciferin. The less rapid decay in Fig. 2c as compared to Fig. 2a can be explained by a lower proportion of the total enzyme level being inactivated as enzyme product complex. In Fig. 2d the addition of both PP_i and L-luciferin results in a stable light emission.

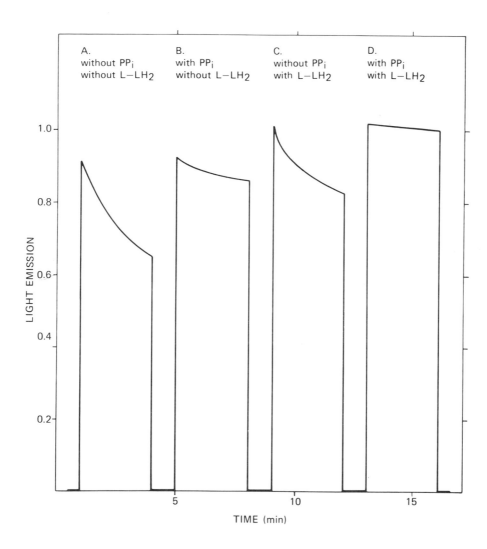

FIG. 2: Stabilization of the light emission in the firefly luciferase reaction by inorganic pyrophosphate (PP_i) and L-luciferin ($L-LH_2$). Reactions were performed in 0.1 M tris acetate buffer, pH 7.75, containing 2 mM EDTA, 10 mM magnesium acetate, 0.1 % bovine serum albumin and 0.4 mM D-luciferin. The reaction mixtures also contained luciferase (C and D twice the amount as A and B), 1.0 μM pyrophosphate (B and D) and 16 μM L-luciferin (C and D). Reactions were initiated by addition of 1.0 μM ATP.

The use of a mixture of D-and L-luciferin in firefly reagents is advantageous not only for obtaining a stable light intensity. Mixtures of D-and L-luciferin are less expensive and have a lower K_m than the pure D-form. Thus a saturating luciferin level is obtained at a lower concentration and at a lower cost. The higher the ratio between the L- and D-forms of luciferin the more luciferase has to be added to obtain the same light intensity. Thus the use of L-luciferin makes it possible not only to optimize the firefly reagent from an analytical point of view but also from an economical point of view.

With an appropriate mixture of D-and L-luciferin a stable light level is obtained within the entire linear range of the assay (<1 µM ATP) provided that degradation of ATP in the luciferase reaction is <1 % /min. The highest luciferase concentration fulfilling this requirement will give the highest sensitivity in the assays. Under analytical conditions, i.e. <1.0 µM ATP, this will result in a production of PP_i and oxyluciferin of <0.01 µM/min. Free PP_i and oxyluciferin will not contribute to product inhibition in these very low concentrations.

REAGENTS

Addition of firefly reagents with a stable light emission proportional to the ATP concentration makes it possible to monitor the ATP concentration in the sample simply by continuously measuring the light emission (19). This can be used for assays of enzymes and metabolites, for monitoring cell lysis etc. as will be described below. An ideal and generally applicable luciferase reagent should fulfill the following requirements:

1) All components for the firefly reaction (luciferase, luciferin and magnesium ions) except ATP should be included in the reagent, since mixing of the individual components before each assay will increase analytical variations and is less convenient.

2) Components not necessary for the reaction, e.g. stabilizers or buffers, should be included in the reagent in the lowest possible amounts, since they may cause analytical interference (e.g. blanks) or may limit the applicability in other ways (e.g. choice of buffer).

3) The light emission should be stable and proportional to the ATP concentration within the entire linear range of the assay, i.e. from the detection limit up to 1.0 µM ATP.

4) The luciferin concentration should be saturating to minimize influence from minor pipetting errors or additions of auxiliary reagents changing the reaction volume.

5) Luciferase activity should be high but should under optimal reaction conditions give a degradation of ATP <1 %/min.

6) Luciferase should be highly purified, i.e. the preparation should be homogeneous and levels of important contaminants e.g. ATP and adenylate kinase, should be low.

A reagent fulfilling the requirements given above is commercially available (ATP Monitoring Reagent, LKB-Wallac). This lyophilized reagent contains luciferase purified by isoelectric focusing (18), an optimal concentration of a mixture of D-and L-luciferin, excess magnesium ions (10 mM magnesium acetate) and for stabilization of the reagent bovine serum albumin (0.1 %). When used in the correct concentration, at constant temperature and under proper reaction conditions as recommended by the manufacturer the light emission is stable and can be used for monitoring the ATP concentration in various applications as illustrated below.

For calibration of firefly assays an ATP standard of known concentration is needed. This standard should contain very little additives and in particular only minute amounts of buffer to avoid that reaction conditions are changed at the addition of this standard to the reagent-sample mixture. A lyophilized ATP standard containing 0.1 μmol ATP without buffer is available from LKB-Wallac.

In many coupled assays based on ATP monitoring with firefly luciferase a pure ADP is needed. Commercially available ADP generally contains a few percent ATP and can not be used in assays of e.g. kinases. However, preparations of ADP with an ATP/ADP ratio $<10^{-5}$ can be obtained by ion exchange chromatography (13).

Assays of ATP in extracts of biological material should be made under reaction conditions that have been optimized with respect to the firefly reaction using a reagent with stable light emission and internal calibration by addition of a known amount of ATP. The buffer should be chosen to give a final of pH 7.75 (pH optimum of firefly reaction) and should accommodate for any variation in sample pH. The luciferase activity in tris acetate buffer (0.1 M, pH 7.75) containing 2 mM EDTA is higher than in most other buffers with similar buffering capacity. The presence of EDTA in this buffer makes it suitable for preparing stable dilutions of nucleotides. Volume fraction of sample should be chosen to avoid a too high inhibition (>50 %) of luciferase activity resulting from sample components.

The assay of ATP as described above using purified reagents with a stable light emission rather than crude reagents resulting in a flash has several advantages:

1) Internal calibration with an ATP standard can be done in each single assay compensating for variations in luciferase activity due to sample compositions or reagent inactivation. Thus analytical interference is easily detected and can generally be compensated for.

2) Sensitivity can be improved by integrating te light signal. With crude reagents only the peak height can be used for analytical purposes (20).

3) Mixing of sample and reagent can be done in any convenient way. With crude reagents mixing has to be done in front of the photomultiplier in order to measure the peak appearing within a second after mixing.

INSTRUMENTATION

The ideal light measuring instrument (luminometer) for ATP monitoring with firefly luciferase should meet the following requirements:

1) A high signal-to-noise ratio for the light emitted in the firefly reaction. Ideally the spectral response should be flat in the region 500-700 nm to minimize the influence from a shift from the yellow-green to the red emission at e.g. acid pH.

2) Temperature control of cuvette (reaction vessel) is needed since the luciferase reaction as any other enzymatic reaction is temperature dependent.

3) Facilities for microliter additions of auxiliary reagents in the measuring position of the instrument. This necessitates a light tight injection channel and stirring of the cuvette.

4) Analog, digital and microcomputer aided outputs are desirable.

5) In the study of photophosphorylation facilities for illumination of the cuvette during measurements are necessary (7).

No luminometer presently on the market meets with all these requirements. In particular a flat spectral response or facilities for studies of photophosphorylation are not available with any instrument. A light tight channel and stirring of the cuvette is available with LKB-Wallac Luminometer 1250 and 1251 only. Temperature control is available with some of the luminometers.

APPLICATIONS

Assay of ATP

The assay of cellular ATP levels require an extraction (release) of the ATP from the cells. The extraction has several objectives:

1) Immediate and irreversible inactivation of all ATP converting activities in the sample.

2) Release of all ATP from the cells.

3) Stabilization of ATP in the extracts.

Previous studies (21) on the extraction of bacteria with boiling buffers, organic solvents and various acids showed that the only generally applicable extraction agent is trichloroacetic acid (TCA). These studies have been extended to algae (11) and recently (unpublished) to various mammalian an yeast cells also including a number of quarternary ammonium compounds and commercially available extraction (releasing) agents. From all these studies it can be concluded that extraction with 10 % TCA should be used as a reference method. TCA strongly interferes with the firefly reaction and extracts containing 10 % TCA can only be used in the assay in a 1 % volume fraction. When a higher volume fraction is needed to obtain an adequate sensitivity in a particular application it is often possible to develope an alternative extraction method using the TCA method as a reference. Alternative extraction methods may involve lower concentrations of TCA, boiling buffers or with mammalian cells triton X-100. The presence of EDTA in extraction reagents inhibits enzymatic as well as non-enzymatic degradation of adenine nucleotides. Furthermore EDTA often irreversibly inactivates ATP converting enzymes during the extraction of the biological sample (21).

Pretreatment of the sample with the ATP degrading enzyme apyrase and triton X-100 selectively lysing mammalian but not bacterial cells have been used for detection a bacteriuria (32). This principle should be applicable also for other samples containing a mixture of cells.

Assay of ATP in an extract of biological material is performed and results are calculated as described in Fig. 3a. If the sample fraction is low (<2 %) and there is no inhibition of the luciferase activity from components in the sample the factor relating light emission to ATP concentration will be the same before and after addition of sample. In this situation (Fig. 3a) it is not necessary to measure the reagent blank in a separate tube, and it is sufficient to calibrate only a few assays in each series of samples by addition of internal ATP standard.

End point assays of metabolites

Any metabolite participating in an enzymatic reaction that can be coupled to formation or degradation of ATP can be assayed using the firefly reaction. In end point assays the metabolite is completely converted to some product and the amount of ATP formed or degraded (directly of after enzymatic coupling) equals the amount of the metabolite. The amount of ATP can be determined by the firefly assay after the end point has been attained. Alternatively the formation or degradation of ATP can be monitored by allowing the reaction to proceed in the presence of the firefly reagent continuously measuring the luminescence. The latter alternative is recommended whenever compatible reaction conditions can be found.

In end point as well as other assays based on ATP monitoring by firefly luciferase the light emission is proportional not only to ATP concentration but also to luciferase activity. Thus the same care should be taken to maintain constant reaction conditions as is done in kinetic assays based on e.g. spectrophotometry. The following recommendations on optimization of end point assays based on ATP monitoring by firefly luciferase can be made:

1) Nature and concentration of buffer should be chosen to be suitable for all enzyme reactions involved in the assay. Since the light

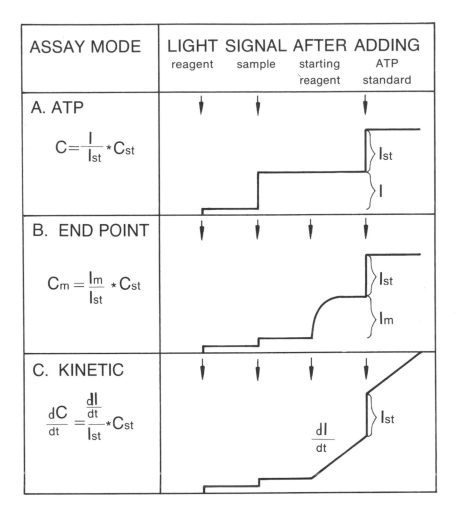

FIG. 3: Assay modes and calculation of results using the ATP
monitoring technique. It is assumed that volume fractions are <2 % and
that additions do not affect luciferase activity. Otherwise it is
necessary to use separate calibrations with internal ATP standard for
the blanks. Slightly different formulas will then apply. In the figure
all assays include the addition of internal ATP standard (final
concentration in cuvette, C_{st}) measuring the increase of the light
emission, I_{st}. If samples do not contain inhibitory compounds it is
sufficient to add internal ATP standard in a few assays in each
series. In assays of ATP (A) the concentration of ATP in the cuvette,
C, is calculated from the increase of the light emission at the
addition of sample, I. In end point assays (B) the concentration of
the metabolite in the cuvette, C_m, is calculated from the increase
(after completion of the reaction) of the light emission at the
addition of starting reagent, I_m. In kinetic assays (C) the rate of
the ATP formation in the cuvette, dC/dt, is calculated from the rate
of the increase of the light emission after addition of starting
reagent, dI/dt.

intensity at the end point is determined by the luciferase activity but not by activities of other auxiliary enzymes the buffer pH should ideally be 7.75. However if the preparations of other auxiliary enzymes are contaminated with interfering agents or are very expensive the assay can be performed at a more suitable pH within the range pH 6-8.

2) Substrates in auxiliary reactions should be added in concentrations saturating their corresponding enzyme reactions unless this causes interference with the other reactions.

3) Enzymes in auxiliary reactions should be added in concentrations so that the end point is attained within a few minutes. Luciferase should be added in a concentration resulting in a stable and high light intensity.

End point assays based on ATP forming reactions are performed and results are calculated as described in Fig. 3b. In this figure it is assumed that the starting reagent does not affect the luciferase activity. If this is not the case separate calibration by addition of ATP standard in absence and in presence of starting reagent should be performed.

Several metabolites can be determined in the same assay by successive additions of appropriate enzymes. This has been exemplified by the determination of ATP, ADP, AMP and cAMP in one assay by successive additions of luciferase, pyruvate kinase, adenylate kinase and phosphodiesterase (19). End point assays based on ATP degrading reactions can be performed in a similar manner.

Kinetic assays of enzymes and metabolites

Any enzyme or metabolite participating in an enzymatic reaction that can be coupled to formation or degradation of ATP can be kinetically assayed using the firefly reaction. In fixed-time assays the amount of ATP formed or degraded is determined by allowing the enzymatic reaction(s) to proceed for a predetermined period and subsequently adding the firefly reagent. In continuous-monitoring assays the enzymatic reaction(s) are performed in the presence of firefly reagent and the rate of change of ATP concentration is monitored by continuously measuring the luminescence. Continuous-monitoring assays are generally preferable if the enzymatic reaction(s) can be performed under conditions compatible with the firefly reaction. Such assays are comparable to kinetic assays based on spectrophotometric or fluorometric monitoring of NAD(P)H conversion but are considerably more sensitive. Since firefly luciferase is added in a low concentration (degradation of ATP <1 %/ min) the luminescence signal is proportional to luciferase activity. Thus additions affecting luciferase activity will also affect the luminescence signal. Such affects are compensated for by using internal calibration with a known amount of ATP.

Optimization of kinetic assays of enzymes and metabolites based on continuous monitoring of the ATP concentration by the firefly reaction is similar to optimization of end point assays (cf. above). However, to get results comparable to e.g. spectrophotometric methods special care most be taken to the enzyme reaction in which the analyte is directly involved. The following recommendations are made:

1) Nature and concentration of buffer should be chosen to be suitable for all enzyme reactions involved in the assay. Since variations in luciferase activity can be compensated for by internal calibration the buffer pH should ideally correspond to the pH optimum of the enzymatic reaction in which the analyte is directly involved. Other alternatives are the pH optimum of the luciferase reaction (pH 7.75) or the over-all pH optimum for the combined reactions. The latter alternative is advantageous if sensitivity is limited by the luminescence intensity and more luciferase can not be added.

2) In assays of enzymes saturating concentrations of substrates should be used. In assays of metabolites a concentration of enzyme giving a suitable reaction rate should be used.

3) Enzymes and substrates in auxiliary reactions (except the luciferase reaction) should be used in concentrations resulting in reaction rates much faster than the rate of the reaction to be measured. Saturating concentrations of substrates is recommended if this does not cause analytical interference.

Kinetic assays based on ATP forming reactions are performed and results are calculated as described in Fig. 3c. In this figure it is assumed that there is no formation of ATP in the absence of starting reagent. Otherwise the rate of ATP formation should be measured in absence and in presence of starting reagent. If the starting reagent affects luciferase activity calibrations with internal ATP standard should be made in absence and in presence of starting reagent.

Several enzymes have been assayed using the firefly reaction including various kinase, phosphodiesterase and ATPase enzymes. However, the only example of an enzyme assay that has been optimized according to the recommendations given above is creatine kinase (Lundin et. al., in press). A routine kit for the assay of total as well as B-subunit creatine kinase activity, of potential usefulness in the diagnosis of heart and brain infarction and of muscular dystrophy, is now commercially available (LKB-Wallac). The analytical performance is similar to the corresponding spectrophotometric method but the sensitivity is much higher allowing measurements of e.g. B-subunit activity in serum from healthy individuals.

In studies of ATP degrading enzymes the ATP monitoring technique is particularly useful since it allows measurement at low ATP concentrations. In this way changes in the K_m value of ATPase in chromatophores from the photosynthetic bacterium Rhodospirillum rubrum could be detected (1).

Monitoring of electron transport linked phosphorylation

In studies on photophosphorylation and oxidative phosphorylation the ATP monitoring technique using firefly luciferase is a convenient analytical tool. Furthermore the sensitivity of the technique makes possible measurements that can not be done with other techniques, e.g. measurements at very low concentrations of substrates or products or using highly diluted or strongly inhibited phosphorylating systems. One example is the measurement of the amount of ATP synthesized after a single flash causing only one turnover of the cyclic electron flow in chromatophores from photosynthetic bacteria (16, 17, 22). Other examples are the measurement of low K_m values of ATPase in chromatophores (1) or kinetics of ATP^m formation after single turnover flashes. (M. Baltscheffsky, personal communication).

Reaction conditions conventionally used in studies of electron transport linked phosphorylation are generally compatible with the firefly reaction. Certain inhibitors and uncouplers inhibit the firefly reaction but this effect can be compensated for using internal calibration by addition of a known amount of ATP. Thus it is recommended to use conventional buffers etc. and compensate for effects on the firefly reaction by internal calibration.

Cell lysis

Measurement of cell lysis by firefly assay of released ATP is an extremely sensitive and convenient analytical tool. The amount of ATP released can be determined after incubation of the cells in the presence of releasing agent. In this way it is e.g. possible to assay concentrations of aminoglucoside antibiotics in serum samples. A sensitive strain of E. coli is incubated with serum for 75 min and then the released ATP is measured by addition of firefly reagent (25). If the releasing time is short (a few minutes) and reaction conditions are compatible with the firefly reaction it is possible to monitor the releasing reaction by performing it in the presence of firefly reagent continuously measuring the luminescence. This has been used for measurement of bacterial cytolysins lysing various types of mammalian cells (8).

Optimization of reaction conditions should be directed towards mild conditions not causing release of ATP in the absence of releasing agent. Such conditions will generally be suitable also for the firefly reaction.

Immunoassays

Any compound directly participating in or affecting the firefly luciferase reaction can potentially be used as a label in luminescent immunoassays. The high quantum yield (close to unity) and the specificity of the firefly reaction make this reaction perhaps more interesting for immunoassays than other luminescent reactions.

Firefly luciferase has been covalently linked to various low molecular weight antigens and such conjugates have been used in competitive binding assays of free antigens using antibodies covalently bound to Sepharose (33, 34). Detection limits around a few picomoles have been reported and 60-70 % of the luciferase activity have been retained in the conjugates (33, 34). However, firefly luciferase is a rather complex enzyme undergoing large conformational changes during its catalytic action (24). This may explain why coupling to protein antigens have not been reported. Furthermore the high molecular weight and the low turnover of firefly luciferase make this enzyme less attractive as a label in immunoassays.

The firefly reaction has also been used to monitor competive binding reactions between antibody, ATP-labeled 2,4-dinitrobenzene and N(2,4-dinitrophenyl)-β-alanine (5). Since firefly luciferase is very specific for its substrates, it is unlikely that the ATP-labeled conjugate was active as such in the firefly reaction. Rather the conjugate was hydrolyzed to form free ATP by enzymes contaminating the crude firefly reagent used in this study. Thus although the specificity of firefly luciferase is in general an analytical advantage, it may impose certain restrictions or additional problems in the use of ATP or luciferin as labels in immunoassays. Furthermore the ubiquitous presence of ATP may cause background problems making pretreatment of samples more complicated.

A very attractive alternative for sensitive immunoassays is the use of ATP producing enzymes as labels. In contrast to ATP or luciferin such labels act as chemical amplifiers resulting in large numbers of photons per label molecule. The technique has been demonstrated using antibodies labeled with pyruvate kinase (28). The ideal label in this technique should be a kinase with a high turnover number in the direction of ATP formation and should not be naturally occuring in high concentrations in the samples (to avoid background problems). For maximum sensitivity a preparation of ADP containing very little ATP is required (commercially available ADP generally contains 1-2 % ATP).

Finally the possibility to measure complement mediated cytolysis should be mentioned. This has been demonstrated both by continuously monitoring the leakage of ATP from erythrocytes (30) and by measuring the ATP remaining in Ehrlich ascites tumor cells (26) treated with antiserum and complement. Potentially it should be possible to design systems for measurement of antigens, antibodies or complement factors.

CONCLUSIONS

The firefly system has a large number of potential applications in biochemistry, microbiology, immunology and medicine. The recent introduction of highly purified luciferase reagents with a stable light emission within the entire linear range of the assay, i.e. the ATP monitoring concept, has further extended the applicability. Furthermore this technique has now become so standardized, reliable and convenient that it can be used for routine analyses in e.g. clinical laboratories. Thus an increasing utilization of this analytical tool can be foreseen in the near future.

REFERENCES

1. Baltcheffsky, M. and Lundin, A. (1979): Flash-induced increase of ATP-ase activitity in Rhodospirillum rubrum chromatophores. In: Cation flux across biomembranes, edited by Y. Mukohaka and L. Packer, pp. 209-218. Academic Press, New York.

2. Bény, M. and Dolivo, M. (1976): Separation of firefly luciferase using an anion exchanger. FEBS Lett., 70:167-170.

3. Bowie, L.J. (1978): Synthesis of firefly luciferin and structural analogs. In: Methods in Enzymology, Vol.LVII, edited by M. DeLuca, pp. 15-28. Academic Press, New York.

4. Branchini, B.R., Marschner, T.M. and Montemurro, A.M. (1980): A convenient affinity chromatography-based purification of firefly luciferase. Anal. Biochem., 104:386-396.

5. Carrico, R.J., Yeung, K-K., Schroeder, H.R., Boguslaski, R.C., Buckler, R.T. and Christner, S.E. (1976): Specific protein-binding reactions monitored with ligand-ATP conjugates and firefly luciferase. Anal. Biochem., 76:95-110.

6. DeLuca, M. (1976): Firefly luciferase. In: Advances in Enzymology, edited by A. Meister, Vol. 44, pp. 37-68.

7. DeLuca, M. and McElroy, W.D. (1974): Kinetics of the firefly luciferase catalyzed reactions. Biochemistry, 13:921-925.

8. Fehrenbach, F-J., Huser, H. and Jaschinski, C. (1980): Measurement of bacterial cytolysins with a highly sensitive kinetic method. FEMS Microb. Lett., 7:285-288.

9. Gorus, F. and Schram, E. (1979): Applications of bio- and chemiluminescence in the clinical laboratory. Clin. Chem., 25:512-519.

10. Green, A.A. and McElroy, W.D. (1956): Crystalline firefly luciferase. Biochim. Biophys. Acta, 20:170-176.

11. Larsson, C-M. and Olsson, T. (1979): Firefly assay of adenine nucleotides from algae: Comparison of extraction methods. Plant & Cell Physiol., 20:145-155.

12. Lee, Y.S. and Crispen, R.G. (1977): Rapid quantitative measurement of drug susceptibility of mycobacteria. In: Proceedings of the 2nd Bi-annual ATP Methodology Symposium, edited by G. Borun, pp. 219-235. SAI Technology Co., San Diego.

13. Lundin, A. (1978): Determination of creatine kinase isoenzymes in human serum by an immunological method using purified firefly luciferase. In: Methods in Enzymology, Vol. LVII, edited by M. DeLuca, pp. 56-65. Academic Press, New York.

14. Lundin, A. (1981): Applications of firefly luminescence. In: Bioluminescence and Chemiluminescence: Basic Chemistry and Analytical Applications, edited by M. DeLuca and W. McElroy, pp. 187-195. Academic Press, New York.

15. Lundin, A. (1981): Analytical applications of bioluminescence-Firefly system. In: Clinical and Biological Luminescence, edited by L.J. Kricka and T.J.N. Carter, Marcel Dekker, Inc., New York (in press).

16. Lundin, A. and Baltscheffsky, M. (1978): Measurement of photophosphorylation and ATP-ase using purified firefly luciferase. In: Methods in Enzymology, vol. 57, Bioluminescence and Chemiluminescence, edited by M. DeLuca, pp. 50-56. Academic Press, New York.

17.   Lundin, A., Baltscheffsky, M. and Höijer, B. (1979): Continuous
      monitoring of ATP in photophosphorylating system by firefly
      luciferase. In: Proceedings from the International Symposium on
      Analytical Applications of Bioluminescence and Chemiluminescence,
      edited by E. Schram and P. Stanley, pp. 339-349. State Printing &
      Publishing, Inc., California.
18.   Lundin, A., Myhrman, A. and Linfors, G (1981): Purification of
      firefly luciferase by ammonium sulphate precipitation and
      isoelectric focusing. In: Bioluminescence and Chemiluminescence:
      Basic Chemistry and Analytical Applications, edited by M. DeLuca
      and W. McElroy, pp. 453-465. Academic Press, New York.
19.   Lundin, A., Rickardsson, A. and Thore, A. (1976): Continuous
      monitoring of ATP converting reactions by purified firefly
      luciferase. Anal. Biochem., 75:611-620.
20.   Lundin, A. and Thore, A. (1975): Analytical information
      obtainable by evaluation of the time course of firefly
      bioluminescence in the assay of ATP. Anal. Biochem., 66:47-63.
21.   Lundin, A. and Thore, A. (1975): Comparison of methods for
      extraction of bacterial adenine nucleotides determined by firefly
      assay. Appl. Microbiol., 30:713-721.
22.   Lundin, A., Thore, A. and Baltscheffsky, M (1977): Sensitive
      measurement of flash induced photophosphorylation in bacterial
      chromatophores by firefly luciferase, FEBS Lett., 79:73-76.
23.   McElroy, W.D. (1947): The energy source for bioluminescence in an
      isolated system. Prod. Nat. Acad. Sci. USA, 33:342-345.
24.   McElroy, W., Seliger, H. and DeLuca, M. (1974): Insect
      bioluminescence. In: The Physiology of Insecta, edited by M.
      Rockstein, pp. 411-460.
25.   Nilsson, L. (1979): New rapid bioassay of gentamicin based on
      luciferase assay of extracellular ATP in bacterial cultures.
      Antimicrob. Agents Chemother., 14:812-816.
26.   Nungester, W.J., Paradise, L.J. and Adair, J.A. (1969): Loss of
      cellular ATP as a measure of cytolytic activity of antiserum.
      Proc. Soc. Exp. Biol. Med., 132:582-586.
27.   Rasmussen, H.N. (1978): Preparation of partially purified firefly
      luciferase suitable for coupled assays. In: Methods in
      Enzymology, Vol. LVII, edited by M. DeLuca, pp. 28-36. Academic
      Press, New York.
28.   Reichard, D.W. and Miller, R.J. (1981): Bioluminescent
      immunoassay: A new enzyme-linked analytical method for
      quantitation of antigens. In: Bioluminescence and
      Chemiluminescence: Basic Chemistry and Analytical Applications,
      edited by M. DeLuca and W. McElroy, pp. 667-672. Academic Press,
      New York.
29.   Strehler, B.L. and Totter, J.R. (1952): Firefly luminescence in
      the study of energy transfer mechanisms. I. Substrate and enzyme
      determination. Arch. Biochem. Biophys., 40:28-41.
30.   Thore, A. (1977): An overview of the work of the Swedish
      bioluminescence group. In: Second Biannual ATP-Methodology
      Symposium Proceedings, edited by G. Borun, pp. 171-187. SAI
      Technology Co., San Diego.
31.   Thore, A. (1979): Luminescence in clinical analysis. Annals Clin.
      Biochem., 16:359-369.

32. Thore, A., Ånséhn, S., Lundin, A. and Bergman, S. (1975): Detection of bacteriuria by luciferase assay of adenosine triphosphate. J. Clin. Microbiol., 1:1-8.
33. Wannlund, J. and DeLuca, M. (1981): Bioluminescent immunoassays: Use of luciferase-antigen conjugates for determination of methotrexate and DNP. In: Bioluminescence and Chemiluminescence: Basic Chemistry and Analytical Applications, edited by M. DeLuca and W. McElroy, pp. 693-696. Academic Press, New York.
34. Wannlund, J., Egghart, H. and DeLuca, M. (1982): Bioluminescent assays. In this volume.
35. Whitehead, T.P., Kricka, L.J., Carter, T.J.N. and Thorpe, G.H.G. (1979): Analytical luminescence: Its potential in the clinical laboratory. Clin. Chem., 25:1531-1546.

Luminescent Assays: Perspectives in Endocrinology and Clinical Chemistry, edited by M. Serio and M. Pazzagli, Raven Press, New York © 1982.

Constant Light Signals in ATP Assay with Firefly Luciferase: A Kinetic Explanation

Karl Wulff, Hans-Peter Haar, and Gerhard Michal

Boehringer Mannheim GmbH, Research Center Tutzing, D-8132 Tutzing, Federal Republic of Germany

The luciferase from the american firefly, Photinus pyralis catalyzes the following reaction:

$$\text{Luciferin} + \text{ATP} + O_2 \longrightarrow \text{Oxyluciferin} + \text{AMP} + \text{pyrophosphate} + \text{light}.$$

The properties of firefly luciferase as well as those of the reaction catalyzed by this enzyme have been reviewed recently (4). Because of the high quantum yield of 0.88 for this reaction (11) and of the high sensitivity of light measurements the firefly system has been used widely for assaying ATP down to concentrations of less than 10^{-13} mol/l.

In many of the earlier experiments ATP assays were performed under reaction conditions where a short burst of light was emitted whose height was proportional to the ATP concentration, e.g. (1). However in 1953 conditions were described under which a fairly constant light signal was obtained for at least 2 minutes at a given ATP concentration (9). These conditions were rediscovered by Lundin and Thore (6) and the analytical significance of this constant light signal was pointed out by the same authors (7).

However, there is so far no definitive explanation for this type of kinetics. There is evidence that the conditions for a constant light signal are not restricted to a highly purified luciferase (5) and that it may require the presence of inhibitors, such as arsenate or other ions (5), luciferin analogs (8) or AMP (12).

In the following investigation we present evidence that firefly luciferase in vitro does not turnover significantly, but rather reacts stoichiometrically with the substrates, forming a dead-end complex with the product. On the basis of this postulate we provide an explanation as to why under one set of conditions a flash-like signal is produced and under another set of conditions a relatively constant light signal is obtained.

MATERIAL AND METHODS

Synthetic Photinus pyralis luciferin (cat. no. 411523) and luciferase from Ph. pyralis, 2 x crystallized (cat. no 411400) were from Boehringer Mannheim GmbH. The enzyme was essentially free of other proteins as checked by gel electrophoresis. All other chemicals were reagent grade either from Boehringer Mannheim or from ^{M}erck, Darmstadt.

The luminescence measurements were made with a photon counting photometer (Biolumat LB 9500; Berthold, Wildbad, Germany). To measure the absolute photon flux emitted by the firefly luciferase the instrument was calibrated using a krypton laser of known energy to excite Rhodamine 6 G and Acridine Orange, resp., in dilute solutions and measuring the fluorescence emission. Considering both the emission spectrum of the dye and the spectral sensitivity of the photomultiplier (VALVO PM 1892) we derived the spectral sensitivity of the instrument being 1 count of the display equal to 2500 photons of the spectral distribution of the firefly emission.

RESULTS AND DISCUSSION

The left part of Fig. 1 shows the typical kinetics of light emission for 1 ng/ml of luciferase and saturation concentrations for all substrates. The same experiment was repeated at 2 and 4 ng/ml luciferase, resp., (data not shown). Extrapolation to t = 0 results in an average specific light emission rate calculated from these three experiments of $I_o = 5.6 \cdot 10^{16}$ photons/min·mg.

Taking in account the quantum yield of 0.88 and Avogadro's number a specific activity of $A_o = 0.1$ units/mg results for the pure enzyme showing that firefly luciferase is a very slow enzyme. Schram and coworkers (10) using a different approach came to the same result.

As one can see from Fig. 1 under these conditions there is a rapid decay of light intensity within the first 10 sec decreasing by about 70 per cent of the initial value. This effect is well known in the literature and is attributed to a product inhibition of the enzyme by oxyluciferin formed in the reaction. The inhibitory constant of oxyluciferin is known to be $K_i = 2.3 \cdot 10^{-7}$ mol/l (2). In an experiment using 2 ng luciferase/ml within the first 10 sec $5 \cdot 10^9$ photons were accumulated corresponding to $9 \cdot 10^{-15}$ mol of ATP consumed. This results in a final concentration of $1.7 \cdot 10^{-11}$ mol/l oxyluciferin. Assuming a thermodynamically controlled product inhibition this concentration should cause no significant effect on the enzyme activity. Furthermore, if the decay in light intensity were due to a product inhibition a second addition of the same amount of fresh enzyme after the decay reaction would not give a significant increase in light intensity. The right part of Fig. 1 shows the results of an experiment in which the light emission was stimulated

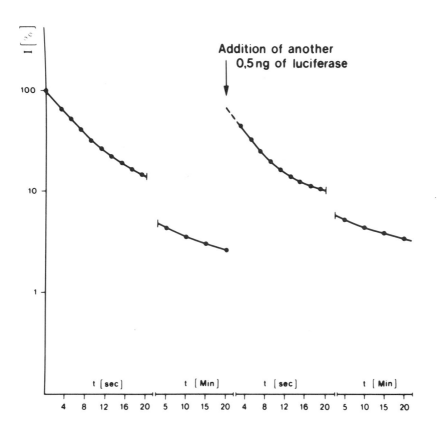

FIG. 1 Kinetics of the decay of light intensity under
conditions of substrate saturation and restart of the
reaction by addition of new luciferase.

The reaction mixture contained in a final volume of 0.5
ml: 175 nmol of D-luciferin, 0.5 µmol of ATP, 10 µmol of
Tris-acetate buffer pH 7.75, 5 µmol of magnesiumacetate,
and 0.5 ng of luciferase. The reaction was started by adding the ATP in 100 µl using the automatic injection system of the instrument. The temperature was 25° C. After a
delay of 2 sec every 2 sec the counts accumulated within
this time interval show on the display. The data are presented in the graph where each value was placed in the
midpoint of the respective time interval. The curve was
extrapolated to t = 0. The intercept on the ordinate was
set to 100 per cent. Twenty min after starting the
reaction it was reinitiated by the addition of another 0.5
ng of luciferase in 50 µl Tris-acetate buffer, 20 µmol/1,
pH 7.75. An extrapolation of the right curve to t' = 0
gives a light intensity of 89 per cent.

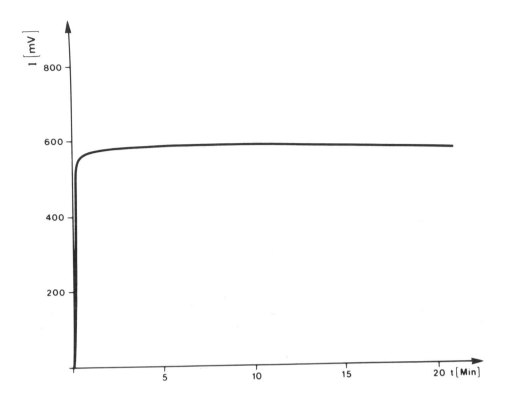

FIG. 2 Kinetics of the light intensity at low ATP concentrations. Buffers and reaction conditions are the same as in Fig. 1 with the following exceptions: 17.5 nmol luciferin, 67 ng luciferase, and $3.5 \cdot 10^{-11}$ mol ATP in a final volume of 0.5 ml. The sensitivity of the recorder output was set to 10^5.

by adding another 0.5 ng of luciferase to the mixture at 20 min. The result shows clearly that after this readdition of enzyme 90 per cent of the original light intensity is restored, which then decays at the same rate as before.

From these data it seems unlikely that a product inhibition by oxyluciferin is responsible for the decay in light intensity. A possible explanation would be that the formation of the complex of E and L in the reaction involves an enzyme conformation such that the dissociation of this complex is blocked. Then the overall reaction would obey the following scheme (E - luciferase in the active form; E' - luciferase in a different conformation; LH_2 - D-luciferin; L - oxyluciferin):

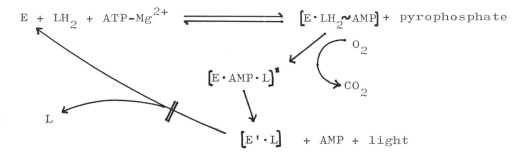

E + LH$_2$ + ATP-Mg^{2+} ⇌ [E·LH$_2$∿AMP] + pyrophosphate

[E·AMP·L]* → O$_2$ → CO$_2$

L ← [E·AMP·L]*

[E'·L] + AMP + light

From our data it may be concluded as a first approximation that luciferase reacts stoichiometrically with its substrates forming a tight complex with oxyluciferin which dissociates only very slowly restoring the enzyme activity.

Fig.2 shows an experiment where a fairly constant light intensity ($7.5 \cdot 10^6$ photons/sec) over a period of 20 min was obtained. From this value an ATP consumption of $1.7 \cdot 10^{-14}$ mol per 20 min can be calculated. The initial ATP concentration was $3.5 \cdot 10^{-11}$ mol/test and the luciferase was $6.7 \cdot 10^{-13}$ mol/test. These numbers predict an 0.05 per cent decrease in ATP and 2.5 per cent in luciferase over 20 min. The decay in light intensity during this time was approximately 3 per cent.

Assuming a consumption of luciferase stoichiometric with luciferin (or ATP) one can conclude that one requirement for obtaining a constant signal is to have a large excess of luciferase present compared with the amount of product formed in the respective time interval of the reaction. In this case the overall kinetics follow pseudo-second order ($v = const \cdot C_E \cdot C_{ATP}$) under conditions of substrate saturation with luciferin and oxygen. From this equation it may be concluded that at relatively high luciferase concentrations the reaction velocity will increase significantly and the rate of light intensity decay will also be greater.

Therefore, the reaction rate has to be reduced. This can be achieved by use of inhibitors, as has been demonstrated by different authors (5,8,12). Under the conditions described in this publication the velocity should be below 10^8 photons/sec·ml. This value may change under different conditions.

ACKNOWLEDGMENT

We are indebted to Mr. Werner Döppen for skilful technical assistance. We like to thank Dr. M. Hauser, Stuttgart, for his hospitality, which enabled us to do the calibration of the Biolumat LB 9500 in his institute. And last, not least, we like to express our gratitude to Dr. J. W. Hastings for many critical and valuable discussions.

REFERENCES

1. Cheer,S., Gentile,J.H., and Hegre,C.S. (1974):
   Anal. Biochem., 60: 102-114.
2. Goto,T., Kubbota,I., Suzuki,N., and Kishi,Y. (1974):
   In: Chemiluminescence and Bioluminescence, edited by
   M.J. Cormier, D.M. Hercules, and J. Lee, pp. 325-335,
   Plenum, New York.
3. DeLuca,M. and McElroy, W.D. (1974):
   Biochemistry, 13: 921-925.
4. DeLuca,M. and McElroy, W.D. (1978): In: Methods in
   Enzymology, edited by S.P. Colowick and N.O. Kaplan,
   LVII: 3-5.
5. DeLuca, M., Wannlund,J., and McElroy, W.D. (1979):
   Anal. Biochem., 95: 194-198.
6. Lundin,A. and Thore A. (1975): Anal. Biochem.,66:
   47-63.
7. Lundin,A., Rickardsson,A. and Thore,A. (1976): Anal.
   Biochem., 75: 611-620.
8. Lundin,A. and Myheman,A. (1979): Germ. Offenlegungs-
   schrift, no. 2 921 975.
9. McElroy, W.D., Hastings, J.W., Coulombre, J., and
   Sonnenfeld, V. (1953): Arch. Biochem.Biophys.,
   46: 399-416.
10. Schram,E., Ahmad,M., and Moreels,E. (1981): In:
    Bioluminescence and Chemiluminescence, edited by M.
    DeLuca and W.D. McElroy, pp. 491-497, Academic Press,
    New York.
11. Seliger,H.H. and McElroy,W.D. (1959): Biochem.
    Biophys. Res. Commun., 1: 21-24.
12. Wulff,K., Stähler,F., and Gruber,W. (1980): Germ.
    Offenlegungsschrift, no. 2 908 054.

Luminescent Assays: Perspectives in Endocrinology and Clinical Chemistry, edited by M. Serio and M. Pazzagli, Raven Press, New York © 1982.

Bioluminescent Method for Determining Microquantities of Glycerol: Application for Measurement of Lipolysis in Isolated Human Fat Cells

H. Kather, F. Schröder, and B. Simon

Klinisches Institut für Herzinfarktforschung, Medizinische Universitätsklinik, D-6900 Heidelberg, West Germany

One of the major difficulties in studying hormonal regulation of human fat cell function resides in the fact that gram amounts of tissue are required for conventional spectrophotometric measurements which can only be obtained by open biopsies. This latter procedure is frequently not tolerated by adult human beings, especially when they are lean, and is almost unacceptable in children. Therefore, sensitive methods permitting systematic studies (100 - 200 assays per biopsy specimen) to be carried out with mg amounts of tissue are urgently required.

Lipolysis can be followed by either measuring the release of free fatty acids or of glycerol. Free fatty acids are reutilized while phosphorylation of glycerol is negligible. Determination of this latter compound is, therefore, preferable for estimating net breakdown of stored triglycerides.

Bioluminescence assays are very sensitive and specific. We thus explored the use of bacterial NADH-linked luciferase for determination of glycerol as an index of lipolysis in isolated fat cells obtained from needle biopsy specimens of human adipose tissue.

PRINCIPLE

Glycerol was phosphorylated to glycerol 3-phosphate by ATP and glycerol kinase. The glycerol was oxidized in the presence of NAD and arsenate to 3-phosphoglycerate according to the sequence glycerol → dihydroxyacetone phosphate → glyceraldehyde-3-phosphate → 3-phosphoglycerate. In standard photometric methods the glycerol 3-phosphate dehydrogenase reaction is driven to completion by forming an adduct of the keto group of dihydroxyacetone phosphate with hydrazine. This depresses the production of light. We, therefore, developed a bioluminescence assay for glycerol which is based on the method of Genovese et al. (1) who introduced the glyceraldehyde 3-phosphate dehydrogenase step, irreversible in the presence of arsenate.

METHODS AND MATERIALS

Needle biopsies were carried out following intracutaneous anaesthesia with lidocaine using needles of 2 mm diameter and a 20 ml syringe containing 2 ml of 0.9 % NaCl. Fat cells were isolated by collagenase digestion (2 mg of collagenase/ml, 45 min, 37 $^{\circ}$C; (2)), washed by low speed centrifugation (3 times) and suspended in Krebs Henseleit-bicarbonate buffer, pH 7.4, containing 4 % (w/v) bovine serum albumin.

Aliquots of the cell suspension (0.05 ml; 200 - 1000 cells) were incubated for 120 min at 37 $^{\circ}$C in the presence of 5 mmol/l of glucose and hormones as indicated in Table 1.

TABLE 1. Effect of isoproterenol on glycerol release in human fat cells[a]

Additions	Glycerol release (μmol/l)
Isoproterenol (10 μmol/l)	6.5 + 0.2
–	2.5 $\mp$ 0.1

[a]Values are means + S.E.M. of quadruplicate determinations. The assays contained 6.000 cells/ml.

Incubations were stopped by boiling (95 $^{\circ}$C, 5 min). The deproteinized media were added to an equal volume of a medium composed of 40 mmol/l Tris-HCl, pH 9.0, 1.5 mmol/l P$_i$, 30 mmol/l sodium arsenate, 1.5 mmol/l dithiothreitol, 10 mmol/l ATP, 10 mmol/l MgCl$_2$, 6 mmol/l NAD, 10 U/ml glycerol kinase, 15 U/ml of glycerol-3-phosphate dehydrogenase, 10 U/ml of triosephosphate isomerase, 10 U/ml of glyceraldehyde-3-phosphate dehydrogenase, and 10 U/ml of 3-phosphoglycerate kinase. After further incubation at room temperature (22 - 25 $^{\circ}$C) 0.4 ml of H$_2$O were added and 0.1 ml aliquots of the diluted media were assayed for NADH.

Luciferase (0.1 mg/ml) and NAD(P)H: FMN-oxidoreductase (1.6 U/ml) were disolved in a potassium phosphate buffer (0.2 mmol/l; pH 7.0) containing 0.4 mmol/l dithiothreitol and 40 g of raffinose. Tetradecanal was disolved in a solution containing 50 g/l of bovine serum albumin and 10 g Triton X-100, pH 7.0, at 50 $^{\circ}$C. Solutions of tetradecanal and of luciferase were divided into small portions and kept frozen at -20 $^{\circ}$C. FMN (5 mg/ 100 ml) was disolved in potassium phosphate buffer (0.1 mmol/l, pH 7.0) and was kept in a dark bottle. The solution was made up fresh daily. The assay contained 0.1 mg of tetradecanal, 0.1 mmol/l FMN, 0.5 μg/ml of bacterial luciferase, 0.04 U/ml NAD(P)H: FMN-oxidoreductase. Portions (1 ml) of the assay were prewarmed at 25 $^{\circ}$C for 20 min. Bioluminescence assays were started by addition of 0.1 ml of samples. Production of light was monitored by a Biocounter 2000 (Lumac, Switzerland) with the photometer settings at "rate."

All enzymes and coenzymes used for conversion of glycerol and for luminescence determination were from Boehringer Mannheim, W.-Germany. Tetradecanal and raffinose were from EGA-Chemie, Steinheim, W.-Germany, and from Sigma, München, W.-Germany, respectively.

RESULTS

Under the conditions employed production of light was linearily related to NADH-concentrations ranging from 0.1 μmol/l - 10 μmol/l. Blank readings averaged 200 - 300 counts when aqueous NADH-solutions were assayed. Inclusion of enzymes for conversion of glycerol to 3-phosphoglycerate was associated with about a 30-fold increase of blank values which was mainly due to glyceraldehyde-3-phosphate dehydrogenase and glycerol-3-phosphate dehydrogenase and is probably caused by absorption of NADH to enzyme proteins. Corresponding to a signal to noise ratio of 1 the detection limit for glycerol averaged approximately 3 μmol/l. Because of the high background levels produced by inclusion of dehydrogenases, samples were diluted 5-fold with H_2O after conversion of glycerol to 3-phosphoglycerate. This permitted the use of small volumes of fat cell suspensions (0.05 ml) during metabolic experiments.

Fig. 1 shows a typical standard curve for glycerol carried out under the conditions finally adopted. Linearity with concentration of bioluminescence was observed throughout a range of 50 pmol - 400 pmol/assay. Duplicate samples agreed within 2 % - 3 %.

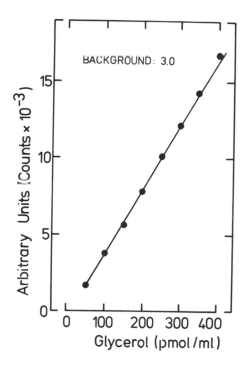

FIG. 1. Standard curve for glycerol
Values are means of duplicate determinations. For experimental details see text.

We used rat fat cells to compare the results of the luminescence method with Boehringer's enzymatic method and found good correlations. There was no significant difference between the methods when tested by parametric and nonparametric tests of significance ($Y = 1.001 - 0.012$; $r = 0.994$; $n = 10$; $p \leq 0.05$).

The luminiscence method for glycerol determination was successfully applied for following lipolysis in isolated human fat cells (Table 1).

Isoproterenol stimulated glycerol release about 2.5-fold in this experiment. Background levels remained constant in spite of a marked increase of glycerol-formation in the presence of isoproterenol indicating that accumulation of phosphorylated C-3 compounds which potentially could interfere with glycerol determinations is negligible in isolated human fat cells under the conditions employed.

DISCUSSION

Human adipose tissue differs from adipose tissue of other species in several aspects. In the rat, for instance, a number of peptide hormones such as ACTH, TSH, LH, secretin, glucagon and parathyroid hormone as well as catecholamines are active stimulators of lipolysis. In aaipose tissue of adult human beings, however, only a single peptide hormone, parathyroid hormone, has consistently been shown to be capable of activating lipolysis. In the rat hormone-responsiveness of adipose tissue is impaired with increasing age and senescence and is markedly influenced by dietary manipulations or endocrine status. Data on human adipose tissue are rare. One of the main reasons for the relatively poor knowledge of hormonal regulation of human adipose tissue resides in the fact that gram amounts of tissue are required for conventional photometric measurements.

Luminescence assays have been proposed for a number of analyses in the clinical laboratory. In most instances these assays provide a rapid, accurate, sensitive approach to the analysis of microsamples for substrates present in very low concentrations. However, application of bacterial luciferase for metabolic studies has been limited until now. The bioluminescent determination of glycerol is specific and sensitive enough to permit systematic studies of human fat cell lipolysis with mg amounts of tissue which can be obtained by needle biopsy (100 - 300 mg of tissue). This procedure is by far less painful than open biopsy; repeated biopsies are, therefore, possible in the same subjects. Bioluminescent determination of glycerol, therefore, offers the possibility of studying the dynamics and flexibility of human fat cell function in more detail. These advantages should be important in elucidating the mechanisms involved in the pathogenesis of metabolic disturbances which are associated with dietary manipulations or endocrine disorders such as diabetes or hyperthyroidism.

REFERENCES

1. Genovese, J., Schmidt, K., and Katz, J. (1970): *Anal. Biochem.*, 34: 161-169

2. Kather, H., Rivera, M., and Brand, K. (1972): *Biochem. J.*, 128: 1089-1096

Luminescent Assays: Perspectives in Endocrinology and Clinical Chemistry, edited by M. Serio and M. Pazzagli, Raven Press, New York © 1982.

Homogeneous Assay for HLA Antigens Using Firefly Bioluminescence

U. Busch, S. Scholz, *K. Wulff, *Ch. Treffert, B. Schiessl, E. Albert, and *R. Scherer

*Immunogenetics Laboratory, Kinderpoliklinik der Universität, 8000 München; *Boehringer Mannheim GmbH, Research Center, 8132 Tutzing, Federal Republic of Germany*

Human leucocyte antigens (HLA) are cell surface structures coded for by a complex genetic system on the short arm of human chromosome 6. These antigens - detected by serological methods - function as the main transplantation antigens, i.e. they are directly involved in graft rejection. Therefore HLA antigens are tested in the selection of donors for clinical transplantation.

In addition the HLA system plays a very important role in the regulation of the immune response, a fact which in man is reflected by the growing number of diseases which show a strong association with certain HLA antigens (such as ancylosing spondylitis with HLA-B27).

For these applications in research and clinical medicine it is desireable to find a test system which is adaptable for automation.

In the conventional assays, the presence of a specific HLA antigen is detected by complement-mediated lysis of lymphocytes which is induced by the specific interaction between an anti-HLA antibody and the corresponding HLA antigen on the cell membrane of the lymphocyte. The degree of lysis in the tested lymphocyte population is determined by staining of lysed cells with eosin or trypane blue.

Since ATP is a major internal component of living cells, its release is a sensitive parameter of lytic cell damage (1). ATP can be measured reliably in the bioluminescence assay (3) which is adaptable for automation. In the present paper we describe the comparison between the conventional dye exclusion test (DET) and the bioluminescence assay (BA).

MATERIALS AND METHODS

The cell samples used for the experiments were chosen at random from the daily samples at the typing laboratory.

The DET was performed in triplicates using routine procedures of the standard microcytotoxicity test developed by Terasaki and McClelland (4).

Bioluminescence was measured with a Biolumat 9500 photometer (Berthold, Wildbad, Germany).

All BA procedures were performed in plastic tubes commercially avail-

able for the Biolumat. In the base of each tube a depression is bored
out to a depth of 0.3 mm with diameter ca. 4 mm. Into this depression
1 µl of antiserum was deposited. To start the immunological reaction,
1 µl of purified lymphocyte suspension was added to the antiserum.
After 30 min of incubation at room temperature, 5 µl of complement
were added and after an additional 60 min incubation at room temperature, 93 µl of an ATPase solution (Apyrase, Sigma) was added in order
to degrade all the ATP released during the reaction. This degradation
is completed in 20 min. Then 400 µl of ATP reagent were added. Thus
in this BA procedure the amount of ATP left in the surviving lymphocytes is measured. Since all extracellular ATP has been degraded, no
centrifugation is necessary to separate the supernatant from the remaining cells.
ATP was assayed by using a reagent kit "ATP bioluminescence HS" cat.
No. 567701, Boehringer-Mannheim GmbH, which was made up to 0.1 % with
Triton N-101 in the final solution. Under the action of the detergent
the lymphocytes having survived the immunological cytolysis become
degraded releasing their ATP spontaneously into the reagent.
All BA tests were done in triplicates. Outlying values were eliminated,
if a significant improvement of the coefficient of variation (CV) resulted from this elimination. This procedure was necessary only in
2.3 % of the 1404 data pairs.
For each cell sample, the results were normalized to a percentage
scale of ATP loss using the reactions with the negative and the positive control sera as references.

RESULTS AND DISCUSSION

In the comparison between the dye exclusion test (DET) and the bioluminescence assay (BA) we tested 54 cell samples against a set of 24
HLA antisera. Together with the positive and negative controls this
results in a total of 1404 data pairs.

Coefficient of variation (CV) in BA triplicates

In 97 % of the triplicates the CV was less than 25 %, and in 75 % less
than 10 %. Correction of outlyers improved these figures to 99 % and
76 %, respectively.

Correspondance between DET and BA

Taking the results of the DET as the reference, we obtained a mean BA
value of 42 % (CV 29 %) for the DET-negative tests and a mean BA value
of 80 % (CV 17 %) for the DET-positive tests. Thus there is a considerable amount of overlap, which is mainly due to the fact that DET-nega-
tives frequently show relatively high BA values. From this it can be
concluded that the BA is more sensitive than the DET.

Variables influencing the BA procedure

The discrepancies between the two test systems are influenced by two major variables a) the test sera, b) the cell preparation.

a) sera:

The sera which are the result of a selection for performance in the relatively unsensitive DET may contain additional antibody populations, which are detected by the more sensitive BA technique. The problem connected with these "false positive" reactions may be overcome by the use of several antisera with the same main specificity, provided there are no false negative reactions. This is a routine procedure in HLA serology.

The analysis of single sera (table 1) shows the variation in the quality of test sera for the BA technique. If no "false negatives" are allowed (sensitivity = 100 %), the predictive value for a positive reaction may be seen to vary between 18 % and 96 %. This type of analysis represents a valuable parameter for the selection of antisera.

It also appears from table 1 that the cut-off point between negative and positive results varies considerably and must therefore be chosen for each antiserum individually.

Table 1:

Evaluation criteria for serum screening.

Predictive value [+] of positive reactions, and cut-off point between negative and positive reactions for several sera at 100 % sensitivity (i.e. no "false negatives").

Antiserum No.	Cut-off point	Predictive value of a positive BA result.
2	75 %	96 %
1	45 %	93 %
10	45 %	42 %
3	5 %	35 %
24	40 %	25 %
6	15 %	20 %
18	30 %	18 %

[+] predictive values (negative or positive) = percent of test results which are truely negative or positive, respectively.

It is possible that some of the HLA-A,B,C sera used in the study contain additional antibodies directed at HLA -DR antigens which are expressed only by B-cells and macrophages. If B-cells and macrophages contain a greater amount of ATP per cell than T-cells (5) (Which is a distinct possibility since B-cells and macrophages have a greater volume than T-cells), then anti-DR antibodies could contribute considerably to the observed "false positive" reactions in the BA technique.

Five of the sera used in this study were investigated by platelet absorption and testing on separated B-cells for anti-DR activity. None of these sera, however, was found to contain significant anti-B-cell activity.

Another possible explanation for the high incidence of "false positive" reactions is the presence of crossreactive antibodies in the test sera. The relevance of such antibodies could be investigated in the reactivity of the test sera with cells positive for crossreactive HLA antigens. Only in three of the 24 sera there was some evidence for the involvement of crossreactive antibodies. These sera reacted in the BA technique more strongly with crossreactive antigen-positive than with -negative cells.

Thus B-cell specific and crossreactive HLA-A,B,C antibodies cannot account for all the observed "false positive" reactions in the BA technique.

b) cell preparations:

Theoretically one would expect that the quality of the cell preparation used in the BA test should correlate with the quality of the numbers. Therefore we investigated the following parameters: cell number, contamination with red blood cells, absolute values of the positive and negative controls. None of these parameters showed a striking influence on the frequency of false positive and false negative results. This does not exclude the possibility that the results could be improved by further standardization of cell preparation.

CONCLUSIONS

The application of a bioluminescence test in HLA serology is described. One important feature of this test is the titration of ATP left in the cells surviving complement -dependent cytotoxicity. Extracellular ATP is degraded using an ATPase which eliminates the need for a separation of cells from the assay mixture by centrifugation, as in the technique described by Descamps (2).

In the comparison of both techniques it can be seen that the BA method reliably recognises the cells positive in the DET. On the other hand, there is a large number of DET-negative but BA-positive reactions. Thus the BA method is far more sensitive than the DET.

The major variable influencing the BA sensitivity was found in the quality of antisera. Therefore sera must be selected for performance in the BA technique. The cut-off point between positive and negative BA value must be determined for each antiserum individually.

The difficult presented by the "false positive" BA reactions may be overcome by the use of several antisera directed at the same specificity, a procedure that is mandatory in HLA serology at any case.

ACKNOWLEDGEMENTS

The autors gratefully acknowledge the excellent technical help by Ms. Cosima Birk.
Supported by SFB 37.

REFERENCES

1. Chapelle, E.W., Picciolo, G.L., and J.W. Deming (1978): Determination of bacterial content in fluids. In: Methods in Enzymology, edited by S.P. Colowick and N.O. Kaplan, LVII: 65-72.

2. Descamps, B., (1980): Determination of intracellular adenosine triphosphate for detecting anti-HLA antibody-mediated cytolysis. Transpl. 29/4 , 295-3o1

3. De Luca, M. (1976): Firefly luciferase. In: Adv. Enzymol. 44: 37-68.

4. Terasaki, P.I., McClelland, J.D. (1964) Microdroplet Assay of Human Seizum Cytotoxins. In: Nature 204, 998-1000.

5. Wölpl, A., Goldmann, S.F., Bribesnecker, K. (1980) personal communication.

*Luminescent Assays: Perspectives in
Endocrinology and Clinical Chemistry,* edited by
M. Serio and M. Pazzagli, Raven Press,
New York © 1982.

Energy Metabolism of Endocrine Cells Monitored by Bioluminescence

S. E. Brolin

*Department of Medical Cell Biology, University of Uppsala, Biomedicum,
S-751 23 Uppsala, Sweden*

In studies of the release of catecholamines from the supra-
renal medulla the concept of stimulus secretion coupling was
introduced (10). It was then surmised that the coupling implies
mechanisms which are interposed between the recognition of a
stimulus and the secretory discharge. This way of looking at the
matter has forwarded progress in endocrinological research and
determined the design of many experiments. Our knowledge of the
events in the initiation of the secretion has been much enlarged
by studies of peptide hormones and membrane receptors. Much attention has also been paid to the mechanisms which effectuate the
final secretory response. Thus, information has been obtained
about the role of microtubules in the transport and extrusion of
hormone granules and about the regulatory effects of ion fluxes
across the cellular membrane. However, it is not clear to which
extent the energy transfer to these processes may participate in
their initiation and in the control of their rates.

PROBLEMS IN THE RELATIONS BETWEEN ENERGY METABOLISM AND HORMONAL SECRETION

Secretory Promotion by Intracellular Factors

Concerning the mechanisms between stimulus recognition and

secretory response, our knowledge is incomplete and fragmentary.
However, the secretory effect of cyclic AMP and the regulatory
role of adenylate cyclase are well recognized (11,13). Furthermore, it has been suggested that the regulatory effects of Ca^{2+}
on the secretion may be governed by factors determining its uptake and intracellular distribution. In studies of the pancreatic
B-cells, experimental evidence has been presented in favour of
this view (19).

It may be near at hand to assume that the recognition of a
stimulus starts a flux of energy which then operates as a couple
and initiates the hormonal discharge. In agreement with this, the
insulin secretion can be raised by several stimuli and each of
them elicits thereby an increased metabolism as evidenced by increased oxygen consumption (17). On the other hand, the metabolism can be stimulated without a corresponding increase in the
secretory rate. The insulin secretion is not raised by glucose
stimulation if Ca^{2+} is absent (19) but the glucose oxidation is
increased (18). Glucose stimulates likewise the glucose oxidation
of the glucagon producing cells but inhibits their secretion (34).

Aspects on Fast Secretory Response and on Prolonged Secretion

How the flux of energy is related to stimulus secretion coupling will remain a fundamental problem in endocrine research.
Connected to this problem other bioenergetic questions will also
deserve our attention particularly when either a rapid or prolonged hormonal release is required. Action at brief notice is a
demand on signal-generating cells which both in nervous and endocrine cells to some extent is met by a store of messengers ready
for discharge. Nevertheless most nerve cells seem to require much
energy and need a continuous supply of oxygen and glucose. In
addition a high activity of adenylate kinase may contribute to
rapid provision of energy by catalyzing direct formation of ATP
from ADP in the reaction 2ADP $\rightleftharpoons$ AMP + ATP. The pancreatic B-

cells possess a high activity of adenylate kinase, much exceeding the corresponding values of parenchymatous organs but still below the activity of certain nerve cells. The A_2-cells show also high values although lower than the B-cells (6). Comparisons with other endocrine cells may turn out to be of bioenergetic interest. However, as pointed out already and demonstrated for insulin secretion, an endocrine cell may attain a high ATP concentration without increasing its secretion. This is naturally in accordance with biological arrangements for the generation of signals, namely storage of energy reserved for discharge of transmittor or hormone granules when required. On the other hand, there are connections between the flux of energy and the secretory rate.

A prolonged and strong secretary activity may be difficult to maintain without cellular damage. In sprayed female rats an increased production of FSH is associated with degeneration resulting in appearance of castration cells and a significant decrease in weight of the anterior pituitary, see Table 1. Likewise,

Table 1. Effect of castration on the anterior pituitary lobe of female rats.

	Weight mg (M ± S.E.M.)	Weight mg (M ± S.E.M.)
Contr.	8.20 ± 0.39 (25)	9.32 ± 0.35 (12)
Spayed	6.88 ± 0.27 (31)	7.14 ± 0.38 (11)

Number of animals are given in parentheses. In the left column the ages at castration and killing were 1 month and 14 months, and in the right 8 and 9 months. The weights are significantly lower after castration (From our material).

thyroidectomy results in degeneration of TSH-producing cells although not accompanied by reduced weight of the anterior pituitary lobe. Long-lasting and strong glucose stimulation of the B-

cells can lead to overwork and cellular degeneration (24). How
the energy flux is linked to metabolic disorder is a physiological question bearing on pathogenetic moments in the early development of endocrine diseases.

APPLICATIONS OF BIOLUMINESCENCE ANALYSES

Preparations of Cell Samples

Bioenergetic studies of endocrine glands are hampered by difficulties in preparing well defined cell polulations (16). Freeze
dried cryostate sections can be used for the isolation of cell
groups. This is accomplished by free hand dissection under a
stereomicroscope. When arranged in layers as in the adrenal cor-
tex the different cell types are well accessible for isolation.
Other morphological patterns have also been utilized for proper
isolation. From lyophilized sections of the rat pancreas the central part of the islets of Langerhans can be removed. Such samples are composed mainly of B-cells since the A_2-cells of this
species are located in the perifery of the islets. Isolation of
the central part of horse islets yields A_2-cell samples of high
purity.

Sampling from lyophilized sections provides information from
the moment when the cells are killed by rapid freezing. Living
endocrine specimens can be prepared by dissection in a cold suc-
rose solution under a stereomicroscope. Pancreatic islets can be
dissected out in this way (14) and reasonably also layers or
lobes of other endocrine organs. Enzymatic degradation of connec-
tive tissue with collagenase (20,23,26) has contributed much to
progress in preparing islets of Langerhans. The insulin producing
cells of guinea pigs can be destroyed with streptozotocin. Islets
can then be isolated which are rich in glucagon producing cells
and compared with normal islets in which the insulin producing
cells are predominating (6,9,34). Treatment with enzymes has also
been used for isolating other endocrine cells.

Contributions of Bioluminescence to
to Micromethods in Metabolic Studies

Preparation of endocrine cells yields often small samples
(16). Most islets of Langerhans are weighing less than a μg,
although islets of a few μg can be obtained from certain species.
However, advanced micromethods have met the demand for sensitivity in assay of such small specimens (12). The Cartesian diver
technique has been developed and refined to permit continuous
recording of the oxygen consumption of single pancreatic islets
(15). Radiochemical methods have been developed and applied for
measuring the uptake of glucose in single mammalian islets and
for determining its degradation products (16). In biochemical
analyses measurements of enzyme activities are facilitated by
product accumulation. Thus, single enzyme molecules catalyze conversion of a great manifold of reacting molecules. This advantage
is lacking in assay of nucleotides and metabolites unless coupling to enzymatic cycles achieve a chemical amplification by product accumulation (25). Alternatively bioluminescence analyses
can be used in studies of endocrine cells since its high sensitivity permits measurements without a preceding accumulation. The
utility of bioluminescence analysis has been well established in
research on the islets of Langerhans. Also, the methods are certainly suitable for studies of other small endocrine specimens
which so far has been found in measurements of ATP.

Analyses of Nucleotides

Adenylates. The pancreatic islets possess a high concentration of ATP as evidenced by analyses of samples dissected from
lyophilized sections from the pancreas (31). Determination of ATP
alone can give some idea about the amount of adenylates which may
be disposable for energy provision. In order to obtain more complete information bioluminescence has been applied for measuring

other adenylates and their sum as shown in Fig. 1. In this study the pancreas of the living animal was pulled out of the abdominal cavity with its vessels intact whereupon a piece of it was cut off above a beaker with chilled isopentane. By the quick freezing the metabolism of the living cells was stopped immediately and thus initial values obtained for the study of the effects of hypoxemia, see Fig. 1.

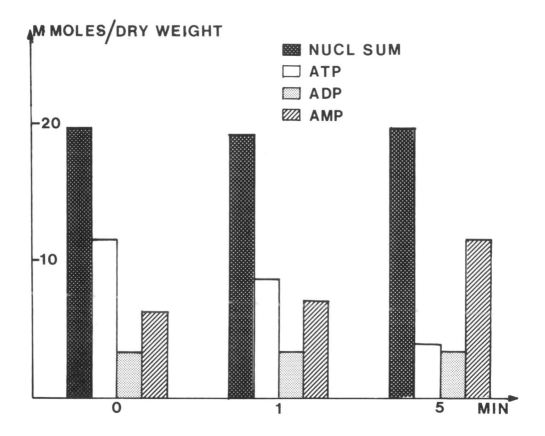

Fig. 1. Effect of ischemia on the adenylate concentrations in the islets of Langerhans of obese hyperglycemic mice. Pieces of pancreas were frozen instantaneously, after 1 min, and after 5 min. The adenylate sum remained unchanged, whereas the ATP concentration decreased significantly. From our laboratory by courtesy of Dr. E. Borglund.

Nicotinamide adenine dinucleotide phosphates. It was early
foreseen that bacterial luciferase could be used for micro assay
of nucleotides (29) but analytical methods for this purpose were
developed much later (3,27).

In islets prepared from fast frozen pieces of the pancreas,
the concentrations of NAD^+ (3), NADH and NADPH (4) have been
determined. A brief period of hypoxemia results in accumulation
of NADH whereas NADPH remains essentially unchanged (2). The
different response to lack of oxygen reflects the main functions
of the two nucleotide varieties, namely rapid provision of energy
and participation in slow biosynthetic processes. The assay of
the reduced nucleotides is carried out in a single step by in-
jecting the sample into a light yielding solution of bacterial
luciferase. When the measurements concern NADH they have to be
proceded by selective enzymatic oxidation of NADPH if present and
vice versa (4). This step may be omitted if oxidoreductases are
used which are specific for each nucleotide.

The oxidized forms of the nucleotides can be reduced prior
to the measurements (3), but again, a single-step analytical performance is naturally preferable and possible to achieve. For
this purpose the light yielding solution is supplemented with an
enzyme and its substrate so that the cofactor nucleotide is reduced. In this way both NAD^+ and $NADP^+$ have been assayed (7,21,
33). A continuous reduction occurs in a cycle which does not result in accumulation of the reduced nucleotide but in production
of durable light emission (33), see Fig. 2. Of course, the cycle
can be started with either or both reduced or oxidized nucleotide. Therefore, the nucleotide sum can be determined as well as
the separate amounts of the reduced and oxidized forms which requires selective destruction of the other. This is accomplished
with weak alkali or acid, respectively as described for analyses
with enzymatic cycling (25). Since specific enzymes are selected
for the continuous reduction, it is possible to measure either
NAD(H) or NADP(H) also when they occur together.

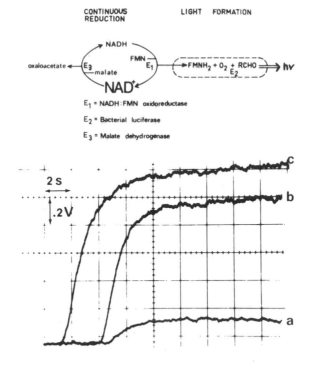

Fig. 2. Light formation from NAD^+. Enzymatic reduction of NAD^+
produces NADH continuously, thereby yielding a long lasting emission of light. In this way a complicated chain of
reactions can be designed and controlled so that a
single-step analytical performance is obtained. The
oscillograms show the light response after the addition
of 1 (a), 10 (b) and 12 (c) picomoles NAD^+.

Analyses of Intermediary Metabolites

It should be possible to measure all substances which can be
converted in or coupled to a pyridine nucleotide dependant dehydrogenase reaction (3). Thus, many enzyme reactions can be
linked to a dehydrogenase step for assay of catalyzing enzymes
and metabolites subjected to conversion. The usefulness of the
bacterial luciferase system for such analyses has been demonstrated by measurements of pyruvates in the islets of Langerhans
(32). Likewise coupling to ATP conversion extends the analytical

applicability of the firefly luciferase system as evidenced by assay of phosphoenolpyruvate in the islets (22). The single-step performance can be adopted for analyses of various metabolites (5,28). For instance, if the cycle in Fig. 2 is modified by increasing the concentration of NAD^+, malate can be estimated. However, this kind of assay has not yet been applied in endocrine research since the present sensitivity is not at maximum. It is dealing with potentialities to bring about analytical simplifications.

Analyses of Enzymes

The low level of detectability makes bioluminescence methods particularly suitable for measuring weak enzyme activities in endocrine specimens as evidenced by assay of 3-hydroxybutyrate dehydrogenase in the islets of Langerhans (1). The convenience and versatility of bioluminescence analyses facilitate also studies of enzymes with high activities. This was experienced in measurements of adenylate kinase in samples from insulin- and glucagonproducing cells (6).

Single-step analyses of enzymes is possible to accomplish, using the principles of continuous reduction as described in Fig. 2. For enzyme assay the concentrations of NAD^+ and the enzyme substrate are kept a few times above their K_M values, making the enzyme amount rate limiting. With this modification malate dehydrogenase is measurable with the system in Fig. 2. However, a meticulous purification of the luciferase preparation is necessary in case it contains even tracer amounts of a dehydrogenase to be assayed. For this purpose affinity chromatography with ciba-crone blue is suitable (8). The convenience and sensitivity of the single-step technique may be expected to be expedient in the assay of enzymes in endocrine glands, particularly when the same kind of cells can only be isolated in small numbers.

Assay of Cultured Cell Populations

Perfusion technique has been extensively used for short time experiments in endocrinology, but preservation of organs by artificial external circulation is difficult to extend over long periods. Small pieces of endocrine gland can be well maintained in culture for much longer periods, provided that the surface for exchange is large in relation to the cellular mass. A favourable surface to mass relationship is a feature of the islets of Langerhans. The culture may improve the conditions of cells subjected to the strain of the isolation procedure. Furthermore damaged cells seem to succumb and disappear in culture thereby eliminating a serious source of error. The condition of the cells can be checked by measuring their ability to maintain their ATP concentration as compared to values obtained after quick freezing of organs in the living animal.

Bioluminescence analyses can contribute information to our knowledge of the relationship between metabolism and hormonal secretion. For this purpose experiments with hypoxia have been designed. It is easy to realize that NADH will accumulate if not oxidized in the respiratory chain and thereby reflect the rate of the oxidation with NAD^+ in the intermediary metabolism. Likewise the rate of ATP formation can be estimated by its disappearance after stopping the oxidative phosphorylation. The redox states of cells can be expressed as the ratio between the concentrations of NAD^+ and NADH and used for evaluations of metabolic changes. This ratio does not reveal which metabolic routes are concerned and does not require corrections which may be raised specifically in studies of the oxidative phosphorylation. In our search for metabolic differences between insulin- and glucagon producing cells the single-step assay of NAD^+ made it possible to evaluate comparisons of their redox state (9). Samples of each kind of cells displayed remarkable similarities, but it remained to be clarified whether the insulin producing cells change their state more rapidly. Close to the isolation the redox state was low but increased significantly after culture, thereby indicating its usefulness in metabolic studies.

Short time incubations in media deprived of oxygen are of value when metabolic studies are extended from determining concentrations of nucleotides and substrates to concern the flux of energy. A perifusion technique has been designed for this purpose (30) and it was found and further sustained by experiments in progress that the insulin producing cells are capable of very fast changes of their ATP concentration.

CONCLUDING REMARKS

In the development of biological sciences we observe how biochemistry and physiology succeed in entering the microscale but this kind of research is still at its beginning and many questions await their answers. It remains to be clarified the extent to which energy flux may serve as a couple between stimulus recognition and the final accomplishment of hormonal release. Increase in secretion and energy flux seem to be closely associated. On the other hand, situations are known where raised energy turnover is not accompanied by increased release of hormones. Among other means to tackle this and related problems, application of bioluminescence may be foreseen to contribute to progress. The analytical experiences which have been obtained in research on experimental diabetes may then be of value in other branches of endocrinology.

REFERENCES

1. Berne, C. (1976): Determination of D-3-Hydroxybutyrate in mouse pancreatic islets with a photokinetic technique using bacterial luciferase. Enzyme, 21: 127-136.
2. Berne, C., Brolin, S.E., and Ågren, A. (1973): Influence of ischemia on the levels of reduced pyridine nucleotides in the pancreatic islets. Horm. Metab. Res., 5:141-142.

3. Brolin, S.E., Borglund, E., Tegnér, L., and Wettermark, G. (1971): Photokinetic microassay based on dehydrogenase reactions and bacterial luciferase. Anal. Biochem., 42:124-135.

4. Brolin, S.E., Berne, C., and Isacsson, U. (1972): Photokinetic assay of NADH and NADPH in microdissected tissue samples. Anal. Biochem., 50:50-55.

5. Brolin, S.E. (1977): Attempts to simplify the analytical performance in microassay of metabolites with bacterial luciferase. Bioelectrochem. Bioenerget., 4:257-262.

6. Brolin, S.E., Wersäll, J.P., and Ågren, A. (1979): Firefly luciferase assay of adenylate kinase in insulin and glucagon producing cells. In: Analytical applications of bioluminescence and chemiluminescence, edited by E. Schram and P. Stanley, pp. 458-466. State Printing & Publishing Inc. Westlake Village, California.

7. Brolin, S.E., Ågren, A., Wersäll, J.P., and Hjertén, S. (1979): Simplified bioluminescence analyses by continuous enzymatic reduction of $NADP^+$ using bacterial luciferase. Ibid. pp. 109-121.

8. Brolin, S.E., and Wettermark, G. (1981): Aspects on the potentialities of bioluminescence assay in cell biology and microphysiology. In: Bioluminescence and Chemiluminescence Basic Chemistry and Analytical Applications, edited by M.A. Deluca, and W.D. McElroy, pp. 287-293. Academic Press, New York.

9. Brolin, S.E., Ågren, A., and Petersson, B. (1981): Determinations of redox states in A_2 and B-cell rich islet specimens from guinea pigs, using bioluminescence assay of NAD^+ and NADH. Acta Endocrinol., 96:93-99.

10. Douglas, W.W. (1968): The first Gaddum memorial lecture. Stimulus-secretion coupling: the concept and clues from ehromaffin and other cells. Brit. J. Pharmacol. 34:451-474.

11. Gerich, J.E., Charles, M.A., and Grodsky, G.M. (1976). Regulation of pancreatic insulin and glucagon secretion. Ann. Rev. Physiol. 38:353-388.

12. Glick, D. (1977): The contribution of microchemical methods of histochemistry to the biological sciences. J. Histochem. Cytochem. 25:1087-1101.

13. Grill, V. (1980): Role of cyclic AMP in insulin release evoked by glucose and other secretagogues. In: Biochemistry and Biophysics of the Pancreatic B-cell, edited by W.J. Malaisse, and I.-B. Täljedal, pp. 43-39. Georg Thieme Verlag, Stuttgart-Thieme-Stratton Inc., New York.

14. Hellerström, C. (1964): A method for microdissection of intact pancreatic islets of mammals. Acta Endocrinol. 45:122-132.

15. Hellerström, C. (1966): Oxygen consumption of isolated pancreatic islets of mice studied with the Cartesian-diver microgasometer. Biochem. J. 98 7c-9c.

16. Hellerström, C., and Brolin, S.E. (1975): Energy metabolism of the B-cell. In: Handbook of Experimental Pharmacology, edited by A. Hasselblatt, and F.v. Bruchhausen, pp. 57-78. Springer-Verlag Berlin, Heidelberg, New York.

17. Hellerström, C., Andersson, A., and Welsh, M. (1980): Respiration of the Pancreatic B-cell: Effects of glucose and 2-aminonorbornane-2-carboxylic acid. In: Biochemistry and Biophysics of the pancreatic B-cell, edited by W.J. Malaisse, and I.-B. Täljedal, pp. 37-43. Georg Thieme Verlag, Stuttgart-Thieme-Stratton Inc., New York.

18. Hellman, B., Idahl, L.-Å., Lernmark, Å., Sehlin, J., and Täljedal, I.-B. (1974): The pancreatic B-cell recognition of insulin secretagogues. Effects of calcium and sodium on glucose metabolism and insulin release. Biochem. J., 138:33-45.

19. Hellman, B., Andersson, T., Berggren, P.-O., Flatt, P., Gylfe, E., and Kohnert, K.-D. (1979): The role of calcium in insulin secretion. In: Hormones and cell regulation, Vol. 3, edited by J. Dumont, and J. Nunez, pp. 33-45. Elsevier, Amsterdam.

20. Howell, S.L., and Taylor, K.W. (1968): Potassium ions and the

secretion of insulin by islets of Langerhans incubated in vitro. Biochem. J., 108:17-24.

21. Hutton, J.C., Sener, A., and Malaisse, W.J. (1979): Biolumi-
    nescence technique in metabolic studies in rat pancreatic
    islets: Practicalities and pitfals. In: Analytical applica-
    tions of bioluminescence and chemiluminescence, edited by
    E. Schram, and P. Stanley, pp. 166-181. State Printing &
    Publishing Inc. Westlake Village, California.

22. Idahl, L.-Å. (1979): Assay of subpicomol amounts of phospho-
    enol pyruvate using the firefly luciferase system. In: Ana-
    lytical applications of bioluminescence and chemiluminescen-
    ce, edited by E. Schram, and F. Stanley, pp. 401-409, State
    Printing & Publishing Inc., Westlake Village, California.

23. Lacy, P.E., and Kostianovsky, M. (1967): Methods for the iso-
    lation of intact islets of Langerhans from the rat pancreas.
    Diabetes, 16:35-39.

24. Lazarus, S.S., and Volk, W. (1962): The Pancreas in human and
    experimental diabetes. Grune & Stratton, New York, London.

25. Lowry, O.H., and Passonneau, J.V. (1972): A flexible system
    of enzymatic analysis. Academic Press, New York.

26. Moskalewski, S. (1965): Isolation and culture of islets of
    Langerhans of the guinea pig. Gen. Comp. Endocrinol., 5:342-
    353.

27. Stanley, P.E. (1971): Determination of subpicomole levels of
    NADH and FMN using bacterial luciferase and the liquid scin-
    tillation spectrometer. Anal. Biochem. 39:441-453.

28. Stanley, P.E. (1978): Quantitation of malate, oxaloacetate,
    and malate dehydrogenase. In: Methods in Enzymology, Vol.
    LVII, Bioluminescence and Chemiluminescence, edited by M.
    DeLuca, pp. 181-197. Academic Press, New York.

29. Strehler, B.L. (1953): Luminescence in cell-free extracts of
    luminous bacteria and its activation by DPN. J. Am. Chem. Soc.
    75:126.

30. Wersäll, P., Brolin, S., Petersson, B., and Östenson, C.-G.

(1981): Evaluation of metabolic rates using bioluminescence analyses. In: Bioluminescence and Chemiluminescence Basic Chemistry and Analytical Applications, edited by M.A. DeLuca, and W.D. McElroy, pp. 287-293. Academic Press, New York.

31. Wettermark, G., Tegnér, L., Brolin, S.E., and Borglund, E. (1970): Photokinetic measurements of the ATP and ADP levels in isolated islets of Langerhans. In: The structure and metabolism of the pancreatic islets, edited by S. Falkmer, B. Hellman, and I.-B. Täljedal, pp. 275-282. Pergamon Press, Oxford, New York.

32. Ågren, A., Berne, C., and Brolin, S.E. (1977): Photokinetic assay of pyruvate in the islets of Langerhans using bacterial luciferase. Anal. Biochem. 78:229-234.

33. Ågren, A., Brolin, S.E., and Hjertén, S. (1977): Simplified luciferase assay of NAD$^+$ applied to microsamples from liver, kidney and pancreatic islets, Biochim. Biophys. Acta, 500: 103-108.

34. Östenson, C.-G. (1979): Regulation of glucose release: Effects of insulin on the pancreatic A$_2$-cell of the guinea pig. Diabetologia, 17:325-330.

Luminescent Assays: Perspectives in Endocrinology and Clinical Chemistry, edited by M. Serio and M. Pazzagli, Raven Press, New York © 1982.

ATP and ADP Measurement in Human Spermatozoa by Luciferin-Luciferase System

G. Fiorelli, C. Orlando, A. L. Caldini, S. Cuomo, and M. Serio

Endocrinology Unit, University of Florence, 50134 Florence, Italy

Adenine nucleotides have been shown to be the predominant nucleotides in mammalian spermatozoa (2). It is also well known that the metabolism of spermatozoa is closely related to the synthesis and hydrolysis of ATP (6,8). Therefore the aim of our investigation was to study the possible role of ATP content in human spermatozoa in relation to the viability and motility.

ATP and ADP sperm content was measured by luciferin-luciferase reaction.

MATERIALS AND METHODS

Human semen from 27 normal donors and 12 infertile men was obtained by masturbation into sterile,inert plastic containers,after 3 days of abstinence. The collection and the physical examination of the ejaculate was done according to the method recommended by the World Health Organization (1). Sperm viability was determined using 0.5% eosin Y (Merck) (1,5).

ATP and ADP were extracted from whole semen,as we did not find detectable amounts of the two nucleotides in the seminal plasma at the same final dilution of the sample.

The semen sample (0.1 ml) was extracted one hour after collection by injection into boiling Tris-EDTA buffer (1.9 ml),pH 7.75,for 5 min. The extract was stored at -4°C and assayed within 2 days.

The reaction mixture for the bioluminescent ATP determination consisted in 330 μl 0.1 mol/l Tris buffer (0.1 mol/l EDTA, 3.1 mmol/l NaN_3, 10 mmol/l Mg-acetate and 0.15% bovine serum albumine, pH 7.75), 100 μl of firefly luciferin-luciferase (SAI,S.Diego,California) and 10 μl of sample.

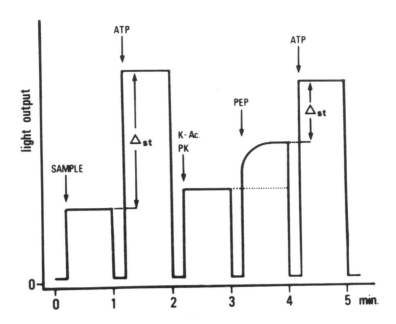

FIG.1 Continuous monitoring of ATP and ADP determination in human spermatozoa by luminescence recording.

The ATP content of the sample was calculated using the internal standard method by addition of 10 pmoles (10 μl) ATP (Boeringher).

   ADP content was measured as the increase in luminescence after enzymatic conversion to ATP (7),by addition of 100 nmoles (10 μl) phosphoenolpyruvate (PEP), 625 nmoles (25 μl) K--acetate and 1 unit (10 μl) pyruvate kinase (PK)(Boeringher) to the same sample. The ADP content of the sample was calcu̲ lated using the internal standard procedure,as previously described.

   In Fig.1 the light output of luciferin-luciferase reaction for determining ATP and ADP in a sample is shown.

   A luminometer SAI-ATP-Photometer 3000 was used to detect the bioluminescence.

RESULTS

   Good linearity between added and assayed ATP was found from 0.05 to 50 pmoles as shown in Fig.2,so as for ADP from 1 to 50 pmoles (Fig.3).

   The within and between assay variation for ATP was respectively 5.2% and 5.1% and for ADP was respectively 8.5% and 9.9%. Good linearity was also obtained in dilution test using a normal pooled sample for ATP and ADP sperm co̲n

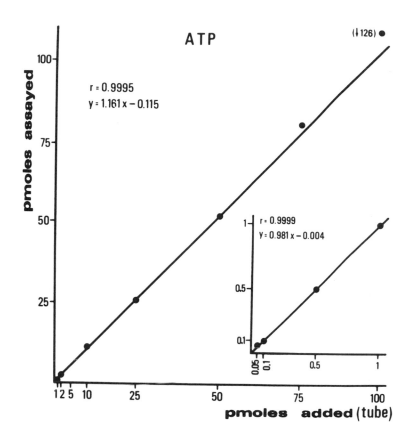

FIG.2 Correlation between added and measured ATP.

tent from 600 to 43000 cells (Fig.4).

The distribution of sperm ATP and ADP content in normal and infertile subjects is shown as frequency in Fig.5.In our subjects ATP and ADP content expressed per 10^6 spermatozoa ranged respectively from 60 to 800 pmoles and from 50 to 500 pmoles.

The wide variation of ATP content found in our subjects was in agreement with the results of other Authors (4,8,9, 10).No correlation between ATP and ADP sperm content expressed per 10^6 cells and per 10^6 viable cells and physical parameters of the semen was found.

ATP/ADP ratio was significantly lower (p< 0.005) in subjects with sperm motility below 50% (Fig.6).

ATP and ADP sperm changes at room temperature within 24 hours after ejaculation was studied in 7 normal donors.At prefixed time the samples were tested for motility and viability and extracted for ATP and ADP determination,as previously described.The results obtained are summarized in Fig.7.

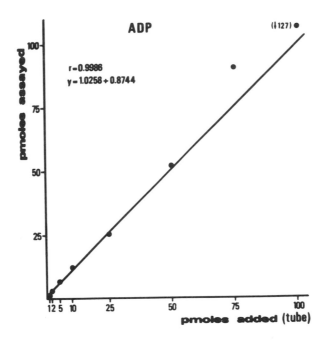

FIG.3 Correlation between added and measured ADP.

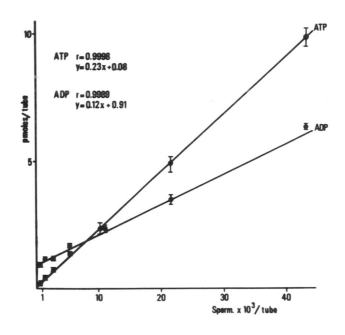

FIG.4 Dilution test of sperm ATP and ADP content using a nor
mal pooled sample.

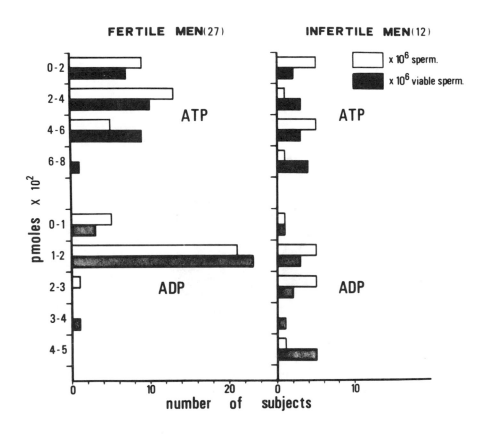

FIG.5 Distribution of sperm ATP and ADP content in normal
and infertile subjects.The white columns represent the frequency of nucleotides expressed per 10^6 cells,the shaded
columns represent the frequency of nucleotides expressed per
10^6 viable cells.

In 5 subjects at the 3rd and 6th hour from the ejaculation
sperm ATP (expressed in percentage of the initial values)
was significantly decreased ($p < 0.02$ and $p < 0.001$ respective
ly) as well as ATP/ADP ratio ($p < 0.05$ and $p < 0.02$ respective
ly).
    ATP/ADP ratio was significantly lower ($p < 0.001$) when the
motility became less than 50% (Fig.8).

DISCUSSION

    The measurement of ATP and ADP in human spermatozoa by
luciferin-luciferase system appeared to be rapid,simple and
to have high sensitivity,good recovery and good reproducibility.
    The extraction of sperm ATP and ADP from whole semen

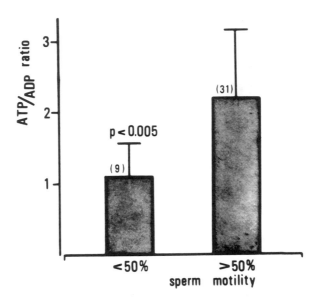

FIG.6 ATP/ADP ratio in subjects with sperm motility lower than 50% (n=9) and in subjects with motility higher than 50% (n=31).

avoided the lack of ATP and ADP due to the procedure for isolating spermatozoa (3). Moreover we did not find detecta ble ATP and ADP amounts in seminal plasma at the same final dilution used in our determinations. The ATP and ADP extrac tion from human spermatozoa by injection in boiling buffer seemed to assure a complete release of the two nucleotides as suggested by the dilution test results.

Sperm ATP and ADP content in our subjects had a wide variation,according to other Authors (4,8,9,10). Moreover we did not find any correlation between ATP and ADP level and sperm concentration,viability,motility and forward pro gression,in agreement with other Authors (6,8).

The significant decrease of ATP/ADP ratio in the subjects with sperm motility lower than 50% seems to demonstrate that it is important to measure the other adenine nucleoti des to investigate human sperm physiology.

Moreover we found that ATP and ADP in human spermatozoa followed a different pathway within 24 hours after ejacu lation,as suggested by the significant decrease of ATP/ADP ratio in the time.

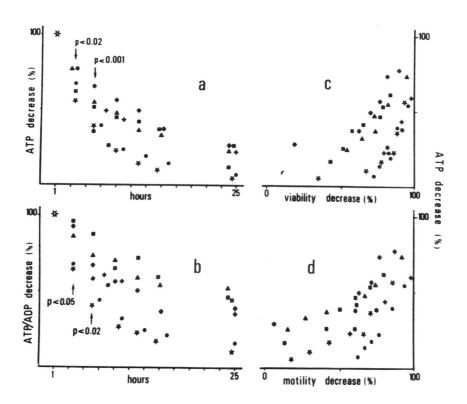

FIG. 7 Nucleotides changes in 7 normal subjects within 24 hours from collection:
a) ATP decrease (%) within 24 hours
b) ATP/ADP ratio decrease (%) within 24 hours
c) ATP decrease (%) in relation to sperm viability decrease (%)
d) ATP decrease (%) in relation to sperm motility decrease (%)

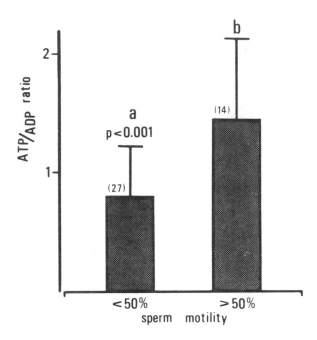

FIG.8 ATP/ADP ratio within 24 hours from collection in 7 normal subjects examined in relation to the decreased motili ty. Column a: ATP/ADP ratio when the motility was less than 50%;column b ATP/ADP ratio when the motility was higher than 50%.

In conclusion ATP content of human spermatozoa seems to be an index of cellular metabolic condition that changes in the time and undergoes individual variations,rather than an index of sperm viability.

ACKNOWLEDGMENTS
This work was supported by a Grant No.78.00447.85 from the Reproductive Biology Program of the National Research Council.

REFERENCES

1. Belsey M.A.,Eliasson R.,Galligos A.J.,Morghissi K.S., Paulsen C.A. and Prasad M.N.R. (1980):Laboratory manual for the examination of human semen and semen-cervical mucus interaction. Press Concern,Singapore.
2. Brooks D.E. (1970):J.Biochem.,118:851-856.
3. Brooks D.E. (1970):J.Reprod.Fertil.,23:525-528.

4. Calamera J.C.,Giovenco P. and Vilar O. (1979):Int.J.Andr.,
   2:225-229.
5. Eliasson R. and Treich L. (1972):Fertil.e Steril.,28:134-
   138.
6. Foulkes J.A. and McDonald B.J. (1981):Theriogenology,
   (in press).
7. Lundin A.,Rickardsson A. and Thore A. (1976):Anal.
   Biochem.,75:611-620.
8. Schirren C.,Laudahn G.,Hartmann E. and Heinze I. (1977):
   Andrologia,9:95-105.
9. Tanphaichitr N. (1977):Int.J.Fert.,22:85-91.
10. Vilar O.,Giovenco P. and Calamera J.C. (1980):Andrologia,
    12:225-227.

Luminescent Assays: Perspectives in Endocrinology and Clinical Chemistry, edited by M. Serio and M. Pazzagli, Raven Press, New York © 1982.

Detection of Cytotoxic Sperm Antibodies Using ATP-Determination: A Comparison with Other Immunological Methods

L. Vermeulen and F. Comhaire

Department of Internal Medicine, State University of Ghent, Academisch Ziekenhuis, B-9000 Ghent, Belgium

Antibodies against spermatozoa are presumed to be the main cause of infertility in about 3 % of barren couples. A correlation between a high concentration of spermagglutinins in serum or semenplasma and infertility has been documented (1, 7, 11). Several methods for the detection of sperm antibodies have been described (2, 4, 5, 6, 7, 9,13). Our study aims at the comparison of the spermagglutinin-test (FRIBERG 2, 4) with a recently described test for sperm cytotoxic antibodies (SUOMINEN et al. 13). Besides, the spermagglutinin-test is compared with a quick method for the detection of IgG class sperm antibodies on spermatozoa, i.e. the mixed antiglobulin reaction referred to as MAR-test (JAGER et al. 8).

MATERIAL

Sixty serum samples from male and/or female partners of barren marriages were tested simultaneously in the agglutinin and cytotoxicity test. Of those sera, 36 were obtained from the WHO Reference Bank for Reproductive Immunology in AARHUS, Denmark. In an additional group of 30 patients, the MAR-test was compared to the spermagglutinin-test in serum.

METHODS

Donor spermatozoa were obtained from apparently healthy men without fertility problems. Motile spermatozoa were isolated by allowing them to swim up against gravity from the semen layer into a layer of EARLE's BBS medium (Gibco 405 S) as described by HELLEMA (3). The agglutinin- and cytotoxin-tests were performed in parallel using the same donor spermatozoa and serum dilutions.

Patient's serum : Aliquots of 1 ml serum for analysis were stored at - 18°C until testing.   Serum was decomplemented and serially diluted in EARLE's BSS medium.

The sperm agglutinating activity in serum was determined by means of the Tray agglutination test described by FRIBERG (2) with minor modifications (8).

The mixed antiglobulin reaction was performed on fresh patient semen as described by JAGER et al. (8).

Cytotoxic antibodies were detected by measuring the decrease in ATP content of donor spermatozoa after incubation with patient serum in the presence of complement (13).   Fresh guinea pig serum was used as the source of complement.   Guinea pig serum displaying intrinsic spermatotoxic activity was, however, excluded.

The cytotoxicity test was performed in duplo : in a first series of cuvettes 40 μl of diluted patient serum to be tested was mixed with 20 μl of suspended donor spermatozoa and 10 μl of complement.   In a second series of cuvettes, diluted patient serum was mixed with donor spermatozoa and inactivated complement.   Both series were incubated during 2 hours at 37°C after which ATP was measured.   The cytotoxicity of patient serum was evaluated from the decrease in ATP in the donor spermatozoa after incubation.   The highest dilution titer causing a 50 % reduction of the ATP-content in the sample with active complement compared to the sample with inactivated complement, indicates the titer of cytotoxicity.

ATP was measured using a luminometer type LKB 1250.   ATP was extracted with Nuclear Releasing Substance (NRS) provided by Lumac.   Fifty μl of NRS was added to 70 μl suspended donor spermatozoa and mixed with 1 ml of 0.1 M Tris buffer pH 7.75, containing 1 mM EDTA.   To this mixture 200 μl luciferin-luciferase reagent (LKB) was added.   Light emission was measured after 10 seconds and expressed in Relative Light Units (RLU).

RESULTS

Technical aspects of the cytotoxicity test

Similar to the results reported by SUOMINEN et al. (13) we found the concentration of complement to influence the cytotoxicity titer.   A complement concentration of 2 haemolytic units per ml of total testing volume is needed to obtain a reliable cytotoxic reaction (table 1).

TABLE 1. Influence of concentration of complement on toxicity titer.

Haemolytic units/	Serum dilution		
ml testing volume	1/32	1/64	1/128
0.4	neg	neg	neg
1	pos	neg	neg
2	pos	neg	neg
5	pos	pos	pos

A higher concentration of complement however reduces ATP causing a non-specific positive reaction.   Inclusion of known positive and negative serum samples in the test series therefore is mandatory.
Some serum samples display intrinsic cytotoxic effect when tested in low dilutions, this effect disappears at higher serum dilutions (Fig.1).

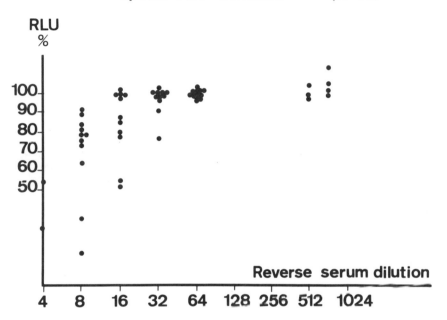

Influence of intrinsic cytotoxicity of serum on sperm ATP-content.   (n = 10)

FIG. 1.   Maximal response in Relative Light Units (RLU) is accepted as
          100 % value.   ATP : adenosine triphosphate.

Since this cytotoxic effect is present in both the mixture with active and with inactivated complement, the difference between the two series remains less than 50 %, and the cytotoxicity titer is not influenced. In sera not containing cytotoxic antibodies, the difference in concentration of ATP between the controls with inactivated complement and the mixture with active complement never exceeds 20 %.

Comparison between different methods :
MAR-test versus spermagglutinin-test.

The results of the mixed antiglobulin reaction and spermagglutinin-test were compared in 30 patients (table 2).

TABLE 2.   Comparison between the results of the MAR-test and the sperm agglutinin test.

n	MAR	FRIBERG (serum)
15	-	-
8	-	1/4 - 1/32
1	+	1/16
1	+	1/64
1	±	1/64
4	+	1/128 - 1/1024

It appears that the MAR-test is negative in 23 out of 24 patients with no, or low titer (< 1/32) sperm agglutinins in serum.   Five out of 6 patients with serum agglutinin titers exceeding 1/32 had a positive mixed antiglobulin reaction (80 % or more of the spermatozoa being attached to the red blood cells).   In the remaining case the MAR-test was inconclusive (between 50 and 80 % of the motile spermatozoa being attached to the red blood cells).   The mixed antiglobulin reaction therefore seems to be less sensitive than the agglutinin test on serum. The former rarely detects sperm antibodies if the serum agglutinin titer is inferior or equal to 1/32.   Most authors however accept a serum agglutinin titer of 1/32 or less to be without pathological significance (12).

Sperm agglutinin test versus cytotoxicity test in serum :

The results of the sperm agglutinin and cytotoxin tests were classified concordant if a difference of no more than 2 dilutions was found between the two (table 3).

TABLE 3.   Comparison between the results of sperm toxicity and sperm agglutinin test in serum.

n	SUOMINEN (serum)			FRIBERG (serum)
	=	↙	↗	
19	neg 19			neg
21	12	8	1	1/4 - 1/32
20	10	8	2	≥ 1/64
60	41	16	3	

In 19 out of 6Q sera both tests were concordantly negative. Out of 21 sera with borderline agglutinin titer (between 1/4 and 1/32)', 12 had a concordant titer in the toxicity test; in 8 samples the cytotoxicity titer was lower than the agglutinin titer whereas in 1 sample the inverse was found. In general, the cytotoxicity test reads similar or lower titers than the agglutinin test in the borderline zone.
Out of 20 serum samples with agglutinin titer exceeding 1/32, 10 yielded a concordant titer in the cytotoxicity test, 8 samples presented a significantly lower cytotoxin than agglutinin titer, and in two samples the opposite was found. Only 4 out of 20 samples read a cytotoxin titer inferior to 1/32 despite an agglutinin titer exceeding 1/32.

DISCUSSION.

The results of the spermagglutinin and sperm cytotoxin tests correlate well, although the agglutinin test tends to read higher titers than the cytotoxin test. It is well known that some non-specific agglutination may occur in the tray agglutination test making the interpretation rather difficult. This phenomenon is noticed in particular at low serum dilutions (1, 2). Furthermore, the clinical significance of a sperm agglutinin titer up to 1/32 is questionable since no correlation with impaired fertility is recorded (12). In the cytotoxin test (13) the demarcation between positive and negative reaction is arbitrarily determined at 50 % ATP-reduction. Using this clear dividing line, reading of the test is simple and unequivocal.
The mixed antiglobulin reaction is a quick screening method for the detection of antibodies of the IgG class on living spermatozoa. This test does, however, not yield information about the concentration of sperm antibodies.
We suggest to screen all semen samples, including those without direct agglutination, by means of the mixed antiglobulin reaction. Only those patients whose semen reacts positive or inconclusive in the MAR-test, should further be evaluated for the presence of sperm antibodies in serum. For the latter purpose the cytotoxin test using ATP as a marker seems to be the more suitable.

ACKNOWLEDGEMENT.

This study was supported by a grant from WHO (core-support of the Special Programme of Research, Development and Research Training in Human Reproduction).

REFERENCES.

1. Boettcher,B. and Kay,D.J. (1969): Nature, 223 : 737-738.
2. Friberg, J. (1974) : Acta obstet.gynec.scan., suppl.36 : 21-29.
3. Hellema,H.W.J. (1976) : Abstracts, 3rd European Immunology Meeting, Copenhagen, 1976.
4. Hellema,H.W.J. and Rumke,Ph. (1976) : Fertil Steril, 27 : 284.
5. Hill,L.A. and Hampton,J.K. (1980) : Fertil Steril, 33 : 302-310.
6. Husted,S. (1975) : Int.J.Fertil., 20 : 113-121.
7. Isojuma,S., Koyama,K. and Tsuchiya,K. (1974) : J.Reprod.Fertil., suppl.21 : 125.

8. Jager,S., Kremer,J. and Van Slochteren-Draaisma,T. (1978) : Int.J.
   Fertil., 23 : 12-21.
9. Johnson,W.L. and Menge,A.C. (1975) : Fertil Steril, 26 : 721-729.
10.Kibrick,S., Belding,D.L. and Merrill,B. (1952) : Fertil Steril, 3 :
   430-438.
11.Rumke,P. (1969) : In : Immunology and Reproduction, edited by
   R.G.Edwards, International Planned Parenthood Federation, London.
12.Rumke,P., Van Amstel,N., Messer,E.N. and Bezemer,P.D. (1974) :
   Fertil Steril, 25 : 393-398.
13.Suominen,J.J.O., Multamaki,S. and Djupsund,B.M. (1980) : Arch.of
   Androl., 4 : 257-264.

Luminescent Assays: Perspectives in Endocrinology and Clinical Chemistry, edited by M. Serio and M. Pazzagli, Raven Press, New York © 1982.

The Use of Intact Luminous Bacteria for Analytical Purposes

Shimon Ulitzur

Department of Food Engineering and Biotechnology, Technion, Haifa 32000, Israel

Luminous bacteria are widely distributed in the sea, either as free living and saprophytic form or as symbionts to marine animals. The marine luminous bacteria belong to two genera, Photobacterium and Vibrio, which are sub-divided into six species. The Taxonomy and the ecology of these species have recently been reviewed (8). The enzyme luciferase, a mixed function oxidase, simultaneously oxidizes the reduced form of FMN and a long chain aldehyde with the aid of molecular oxygen. The products of the reaction are: Light, FMN; H_2O and a long chain fatty acid. (5, 8).

The analytical applications of the bacterial luminescence system has recently been reviewed by several authors (3,13,29). Almost all the analytical applications described so far are based on the luminescence system of the cell-free extracts, the use of the whole, intact luminous bacteria for analytical purposes has been almost completely ignored. This field has only recently been explored and will be discussed in some detail in this communication.

The use of the whole intact luminous bacteria for analytical purposes has some clear advantages: The intact luminous bacterium is a self-maintaining luminescence unit, that, under proper conditions, emits a high and steady level of luminescence. The light of a single bacterium may reach 5×10^4 quanta·sec^{-1}·$cell^{-1}$, a level that can be readily determined with the aid of a photoncounter (22), while the luminescence of a bacterial suspension consisting of only a few hundred cells per milliliter can be determined by almost any simple photometer.

Growing and handling luminous bacteria, that are non-pathogenic, is very simple and requires no special equipment or technical skill. Moreover, the luminous bacteria may be lyophilized and stored for many months in a cold room. Such lyophilized cultures promptly resume their full level of in vivo luminescence upon rehydration.

From the analytical point of view the intact luminous bacteria can be used as a probe for determining the activity of various physico-

chemical factors that may affect cell integrity or different levels in
the bacterial metabolism. The analytical applications using intact
luminous cells have been developed along three main lines:

The first approach is to use the luminous bacteria as a "sac of
enzymes" in which we control the concentration or the activity of any
desired component. This task can be performed by using a proper bacterial mutant which lacks a certain activity required for the functioning
of the luminescence system. Mutants that require myristic acid (the precursor of the intrinsic aldehyde) or long-chain aldehyde are very dim
unless supplied by an external source of these components. As will be
described later, such mutants are used for assaying picomole amounts of
aldehydes or long-chain fatty acids, and serve as a basis for sensitive
assays for different lipolytic enzymes, as well as for other tests. The
oxygen is another component of the luminescence system whose concentration in the solution can be easily controled. Luminous bacteria were
applied for determination of very low concentration of O_2(10). An adenosine 3'.5'-cyclic monophosphate(cAMP) requiring mutant of luminous
bacteria was used to detect as low as 5 ng of cAMP (14).

The second approach in using luminous bacteria as an analytical tool
is to assess the effect of different physico-chemical or biological
factors on the formation or the activity of the luminescence system in
the intact luminous bacteria.

Different antimicrobial agents, including antibiotics of different
kinds, inhibit the synthesis of luciferase or affect cell integrity.
Most of these agents can be assayed by a procedure which lasts less than
one hour. Some tests for antibiotics will be described. The whole
luminous cell can also be used as a non-specific sensor, assaying different toxic substances in the environment. This principle was used for
detecting polluted air(11), and anaesthetics (4,6,7,12) and has recently
been used for evaluating water quality (1,27).

Another biological system that could be monitored with the aid of
luminous bacteria is the bactericidal activity of the biological fluids.
The kinetics of luminous bacteria digestion by polymorphonuclear phagocytes or the rate of lysis of luminous bacteria by the immunoglobulins-
complement system of the serum can easily be followed. The analytical
applications of these systems will be described.

The third approach is to use the luminous bacteria as an object for
evaluation of the activity of mutagenic and carcinogenic agents on the
microbial genome. This test is based upon the ability of a chemical to
alter physically or chemically the DNA of a certain dark variant of
luminous bacteria. Such alteration in the DNA structure or composition
results in restoration of the capacity of the cells to synthetize luciferase and to emit light. As will be described, it is possible to detect
nanogram quantities of different kinds of carcinogenic agents by a simple
non-expensive, fast and almost completely automatic procedure.

The following sections will describe in some detail the different
bioassays that were developed in our laboratory and will discuss their
potential use in clinical chemistry.

BIOLUMINESCENCE ASSAYS THAT USE FATTY ACIDS AND ALDEHYDE DEPENDENT
LUMINESCENT BACTERIAL MUTANTS.

Ulitzur and Hastings (19,20,21) have shown that certain dim
"aldehyde" mutants of luminous bacteria respond not only to long-chain
aldehydes but also to some long chain fatty acids, especially to myristic
acid. Under proper conditions, as low as 10 p moles of myristic acid and
100-200 p moles of oleic and palmitic acids as well as long-chain aldehydes can easily be detected within a few seconds. It is evident, therefore, that one could thereby determine any hydrolytic or enzymatic activity that will liberate aldehydes or fatty acids, especially myristic
acid, from a complex lipid. Using commercially available substrates,
such as trimyristin or L-α-dimyristoyl phosphatidyl-choline, one can assay
low concentrations of lipase, phospholipase A_2 and phospholipase-C,
(15,16,17,23). For phospholipase C, the detection is based on a coupled
assay, in which the mixture contains an excess of lipase which immediately hydrolyzes the diglyceride formed. The assays may be run continuously where the enzyme which is being assayed, the substrate and the
bacteria are all incubated together and the kinetics of the reaction are
followed graphically. Alternatively, the hydrolytic stage may be carried
out separately and it is then followed by the independent assays of the
products. In addition to these lipolytic enzymes, one can use these
mutants to detect other hydrolytic enzymes that liberate myristic acid
or long-chain aldehydes. This group includes enzymes such as esterase
(using myristic acid ethyl ester as a substrate) and serum choline-
esterase (using myristoyl-choline as a substrate). Enzymes that hydro-
lyze plasmologens can be determined with the aid of aldehyde-requiring
mutants. Compounds rich in myristic acid or long chain aldehydes can
also be determined with these mutants. One of the components which is
rich in myristic acid is lipopolysaccharide (LPS), the endotoxin of
Gram negative bacteria. Ulitzur et al (19) have shown that as little as
50 ng of LPS can be determined with the aid of the myristic acid requiring mutant. The same assay is also applied for estimating the total
number of Gram negative bacteria in water. For this purpose the myristic
acid is liberated from the cells by weak alkali hydrolysis. We have
found (unpublished observation) that as few as 10^5 cells·ml^{-1} of different Gram negative bacteria can be determined by such bioluminescence test.

As we have recently shown (25), long-chain unsaturated fatty acids
such as oleic, linoleic or palmitoleic acids are strong inhibitors of the
myristic acid initiating luminescence. Since the degree of inhibition is
proportional to the concentration of the unsaturated fatty acids, one can
use this system for the determination of nano moles amounts of these unsaturated fatty acids. To overcome the strong inhibition by the unsaturated fatty acids, the samples should be treated with bromine followed
by an addition of thiosulfate. The difference in luminescence before and
after the bromination is directly related to the concentration of the unsaturated fatty acids in the sample (paper in preparation).

Aldehyde mutants of luminous bacteria can also be used in the determination of NAD^+ or $NADH_2$. The assay uses the enzyme horse liver alcohol
dehydrogenase which is incubated with ethanol (in excess) and long chain
aldehyde in the presence of NAD^+ or $NADH_2$. The alcohol dehydrogenase
generates $NADH_2$ by ethanol oxidation and uses it to reduce the long chain

aldehyde to the corresponding alcohol. Neither acetaldehyde nor the
long chain alcohol are active in the production of light by these mutants.

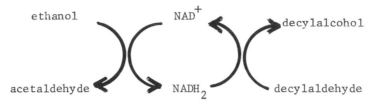

Using this assay it is possible within a 5 minute procedure, to detect
as little as 10^{-10}M NAD$^+$ (Fig. 1.) As we have recently shown in this
assay a lyophilized culture of aldehyde-requiring strain of luminous
bacteria can be used.

FIG. I: DETERMINATION OF NAD$^+$ BY ALDEHYDE REQUIRING
          MUTANT OF LUMINOUS BACTERIA.

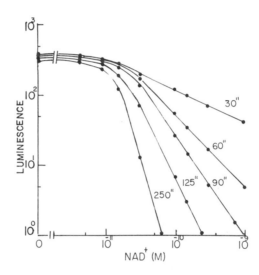

*The aldehyde requiring mutant of Photobacterium fischeri AD-23 was
grown in ASWRP liquid medium (24) to an optical density of 0.35 OD 660.
The culture was kept in ice until required. NAD$^+$ was added at different concentrations to 1 ml MOPS buffer (0.02M pH-7.0) containing 10μg
horse liver alcohol dehyrodegenase (E.C.1.1.1.1) and 10μl of ethanolic
solution of tetradecanal (50 μM) (final concentrations: ethanol - 1% and
tetradecanal: 0.5 μM). The mixture was incubated at 35°C for different
intervals. To determine the aldehyde concentration, 0.2 ml samples were
added to 1 ml of the aldehyde requiring mutant culture at 25°C and the
maximal in vivo luminescence was recorded. The figure shows the maximal
luminescence obtained after incubations of the mixture for the periods
that are shown in the figure (in seconds).*

SHORT-TERM BACTERIAL BIOLUMINESCENCE TESTS FOR ANTIBIOTICS

Short term tests for antibiotics are mainly required to determine the momentary concentration of the antibiotic in biological fluids such as milk, urine or blood. In medicine, great importance is placed on determining the momentary concentration of some antibiotics such as gentamicin in serum.

The shortest known assay for gentamicin (or other antibiotics) was developed by Nillson (9) and others (2). This test determines the cellular residual ATP or the ATP which leaks from the antibiotic treated bacterial cultures. However these tests still require about 3 hours. The minimal detected concentrations of gentamicin in these tests is about 1-2 μg.ml^{-1}.

The new bacterial bioluminescence tests for antibiotics are much more sensitive and shorter than the above mentioned tests. The new tests are based on three different principles. The first test, "The Lysis-Test" uses a sensitive, highly luminescent culture of luminous bacteria. In the presence of antibiotics that affect cell integrity, luminescence falls drastically. Using this system, we were able to detect 0.01μg.ml^{-1} of polymyxin-B and E in a very short procedure (Ulitzur in preparation). The use of certain rough mutants of luminous bacteria or spheroplasts of these cells makes it possible to increase the sensitivity of the assay. As a control for this and other antibiotics assays, we used a selected antibiotic resistant mutant of luminous bacteria, which is relatively resistant to the tested antibiotic. This allows determination of the desired antibiotic compound in the presence of other antibiotics. In principle, this test may be applied for testing penicillins and different β-lactams as well. However, being Gram negative, the luminous bacteria are relatively stable to these kinds of antibiotics. A deep rough mutant of luminous bacteria was found to show higher sensitivity to these antibiotics.

To test the antibiotics that act at the level of protein synthesis, two other tests were applied by Naveh and Ulitzur (in preparation). The first one ("Induce-Test") is based on the ability of the tested antibiotic to inhibit the luciferase synthesis in the treated cells. For this test we use a specific dark variant of luminous bacteria that undergoes prompt induction in the presence of certain DNA intercalating agents, such as norharman or acridine dyes (24,26). The *in vivo* luminescence of the acridine-treated cells increases more than 30 fold within 30 minutes. This increase in the *in vivo* luminescence is highly sensitive to the presence of very low concentrations of certain antibiotics (Fig 2).

The second test uses a biological coupled system in which highly luminescent bacteria are mixed with a specific bacterio-phage (Phage-Test). In the absence of the antibiotic, the luminous bacteria are lysed within 45 minutes and their *in vivo* luminescence drops to almost zero. Antibiotics that inhibit DNA, RNA or protein synthesis, also inhibit the intracellular phage development and thus save the luminous bacteria.

The minimal concentrations of antibiotics that are detectable in these tests are 0.05 μg·ml^{-1} chloramphenicol, 0.2 μg·ml^{-1} gentamicin, kanamycin or streptomycin and 1-2 μg·ml of tetracycline. With the "Phage

FIG.2 :   <u>DETERMINATION OF GENTAMICIN IN SERUM WITH</u>
<u>LUMINOUS BACTERIA</u>

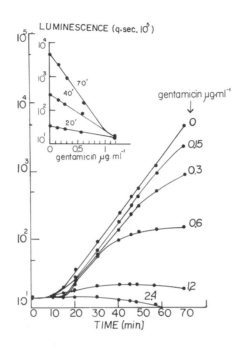

Gentamicin was added at different concentrations to
a set of vials containing each one ml samples of pooled
human serum that was adjusted to pH 8.0 with NaOH.   The
bactericidal activity of the serum was inactivated by
thermal treatment (70°C, 5 min.).   To each vial, 0.1 ml
of the   inducer norharman (2.5mg/ml) and 0.1 ml of
a logarithmic culture(10⁸ cells per ml) of the dark
variant <u>Photobacterium leiognathi</u> 8SD18 (28) were
added.   The vials were incubated in temperature controled scintillation counter and the luminescence was
recorded repeatedly.   The figure shows the luminescence
in vials containing various concentrations of gentamicin.
The insert presents the correlation between the gentamicin
concentration and the luminescence after 20, 40 and 70
minutes of incubation at 30°C.

Test" one can detecl also the DNA synthesis inhibitors: Novobiocin,
nalidixic acid etc.

The main advantages of the new bioluminescence tests are:
1) The tests are very sensitive and fast (the whole procedure takes

only 30-45 minutes); 2) The tests are specific and determine the activity of the tested antibiotic as DNA, RNA or protein synthesis inhibitors; 3) The tests are very economical, simple and can be run automatically; 4) The minimal volume required for these tests is 0.1 ml or even less; 5) It is possible to use a strain resistant to certain antibiotics and to determine specifically the action of mixtures of antibiotics. In order to determine the antibiotics in serum, one should first neutralize the bactericidal activity of the serum due to the activity of the immunological proteins and the complement system (see below). These bactericidal activities can be easily eliminated by pre-incubation of the serum at 70°C for 5 minutes. To determine the activity of the aminoglycosides antibiotics the pH of the serum is preferably increased to 8.0, (see Fig. 2).

THE USE OF LUMINOUS BACTERIA FOR THE DETERMINATION OF PHAGOCYTOSIS

The existing short-term methods for phagocytosis evaluation are limited by the fact that none of these tests determine the real events occurring during phagocytosis of microorganisms. Moreover, the individual tests do not allow a continuous determination of the kinetics of the process. By using luminous bacteria as an object for phagocytosis one can easily determine the kinetics of the process by following the rate of decrease in the luminescence of the bacteria due to their ingestion by the phagocytes. Barak & Ulitzur have recently shown (paper in preparation) that the terrestrial luminous bacteria Vibrio cholerae (var. albensis) are phagocytized and there is a direct correlation between the level of their in vivo luminescence and viability (see Fig. 3). In order to achieve maximal phagocytosis rate, opsonization by 5-10% serum is required. Thermally-inactivated (56°C, 30 min) serum does not potentiate the process. This test can replace the commonly used bactericidal test for clinical determination of phagocytic and opsonic abilities of phagocytes and serum from different sources (e.g., neonates, chronic granulomatous disease (CGD), neoplastic diseases etc).

The bioluminescence test can also be used as a model for studying the influence of different biological and physicochemical factors on the kinetics of phagocytosis.

THE USE OF LUMINOUS BACTERIA FOR DETERMINATION OF THE SERUM BACTERICIDAL ACTIVITY.

Non-marine luminous bacteria belonging to the genus Vibrio cholerae are extremely sensitive to the bactericidal activity of human serum. Luminous bacteria incubated in a buffer containing 10% or more serum undergo lysis, accompanied by a corresponding decrease in luminescence. The decrease in the in vivo luminescence is proportional to the decrease in the viable count and is a function of the serum concentration. The bacteriolytic activity of the serum was found to be due to the presence of immunoglobulins and the complement system. Serum lacking immunoglobulins (adsorbed on killed bacteria)or certain complement components, especially C_3,does not affect the luminescence (Fig. 4). As found in other systems, the bacteriolytic activity of the serum is only potentiated

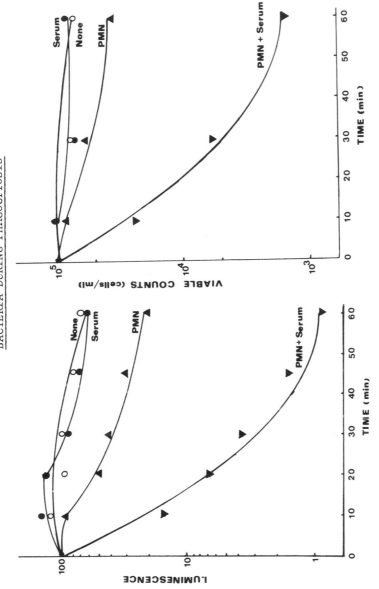

FIG. 3: LUMINESCENCE AND VIABLE COUNT OF LUMINOUS BACTERIA DURING PHAGOCYTOSIS

Luminous Vibrio cholerae cells were grown with shaking in nutrient broth containing 1% NaCl at 37°C. Late logarithmic phase culture (1.10^9 cells $\times$ ml^{-1}) was diluted to a final concentration of 10^7 cells per ml in saline without or with 5% pooled human serum. Dextrose separated leucocytes were adjusted to 10^7 cells per ml. The assay system consists of 0.1 ml luminous bacteria; 0.5 ml leucocytes and 0.4 ml HBSS buffer. The vials were incubated with moderate shaking at 37°C and the in vivo luminescence and bacterial viable count were determined with time.

FIG. 4: THE EFFECT OF VARIOUS COMPONENTS OF HUMAN SERUM
ON THE IN VIVO LUMINESCENCE OF V. CHOLERAE.

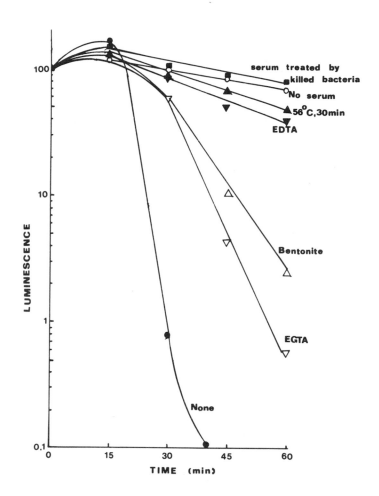

$V.$ $cholerae$ cells (10^7 cells/ml) (see Fig. 3) were suspended in
one $\underline{ml}$ of PBS with 10mM glucose and 0.1% BSA containing 30%
pooled human serum. The sera samples were subjected to the
following treatments: 1) Thermal inactivation of the complement
system (56°C, 30 min). 2) Immunoglobulins adsorption by 10^8
heat killed luminous bacteria. 3) Lysozyme adsorption by bento-
nite (3 mg/ml). 4) Addition of EDTA (10 mM). 5) Addition of
Mg-EGTA (10 mM). The samples were shaken at 37°C and the $\underline{in}$-
$\underline{vivo}$ luminescence was determined with time.

FIG. 5:   EFFECT OF COMPLEMENT COMPONENTS DEFICIENCIES
          ON THE LUMINESCENCE OF V. CHOLERAE CELLS.

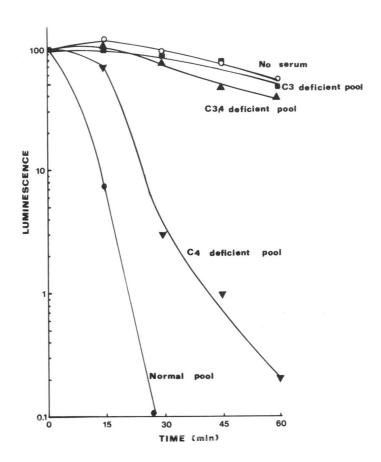

V. cholerae (10^7 cells/ml) were suspended in 30% human sera
from the following sources: 1)   Pooled normal serum;   2) Pooled
C-3 deficient serum;   3)   Pooled *C-4* deficient serum;   4)   Serum
deficient in both *C3* and *C4*.   The samples were incubated at $37^{\circ}C$
with shaking and the luminescence was determined with time.

by lyzozyme, but it is not lyzozyme-dependent. As shown (see Fig.4), this system can easily distinguish between C' classical pathway and the properdin pathway. EGTA, which inhibits only the classical C' pathway, does not inhibit the decrease in luminescence as does EDTA, indicating that the properdin pathway is very active.

This fact enables one to distinguish between deficiencies in C' components participating in both pathways as C_3, and C' components, that are involved only in the classical pathway, as does C_4 (Fig. 5). Thus, this system can be applied for determining deficiencies of certain complement components, as well as an alternative to the hemolytic system in the complement fixation tests. Complement fixation tests using luminous bacteria for detection of influenza and syphilis antibodies, were found to be at least twice as sensitive as the same tests using the hemolytic system (Barak & Ulitzur in preparation).

THE USE OF BACTERIA FOR DETECTION OF MUTAGENIC AND CARCINOGENIC AGENTS

There is increasing evidence that the initiation of human cancer involves mutational events. This has led to the concept that mutagenic chemicals are also likely to be carcinogenic. Therefore, tests for chemical mutagenicity might reveal their carcinogenic potential. Based on this concept we have recently developed new, fast and sensitive bio-luminescence assays for testing mutagenic potential of different chemical agents (24,26, 28). The suggested test uses a stable dark variant of luminous bacteria, and determines the ability of different agents to restore the luminescent state.

The inability of the dark variant to emit light seems to stem from the high repression state of the luciferase cistron. Restoration of the luminescence of the dark variant cells could theoretically be achieved by three independent events: (1) Blocking of the formation of the repressor, thus altering the repressors' or the operons' sites structure; (2) Changing the configuration of the DNA structure, thus allowing unrepressed transcription of the luciferase operon; (3) Inactivation of the repressor of the luminescence system. These events seem to occur under the influence of three different groups of chemical agents,(Table 1).

1) Direct mutagens: The members of this group include base-substitution and frame-shift agents, are active at very low concentrations, and bring about the formation of stable luminous forms. These agents are supposed to act either on the formation of the repressor of the luminescence system, or by altering its ability to bind to the operon site (24).

2) DNA-intercalating agents: This group includes organic chemicals that are capable of intercalating between the DNA bases, resulting in formation of a relaxation state of the DNA. When the DNA intercalating agents are covalently bound to the DNA, it may lead to a frame-shift mutation that may initiate carcinogenic event. All the DNA intercalating agents so far tested are highly active in restoring the in vivo luminescence in the dark variant cells. These agents act almost promptly (within 10 minutes) and restore almost completely the in vivo luminescence in the treated cells. However, in spite of the high level of in vivo luminescence, no stable genetic forms were found.

Table 1 : The minimal concentrations of different mutagens that are significantly detected by the Bioluminescence-Test .

(1) Base-substitution agents	$\mu g \cdot ml^{-1}$
N-Methyl-N-nitro-N-nitrosoguanidine (NTG)	0.002
Ethyl methan sulfonate (EMS)	0.005
Hydroxylamine (HA)	0.1
Hydrazine	0.07
(2) Frame-shift agents	
4-nitroquinoline-N-oxide	0.6
20 methyl cholanthrene (*)	1.0
Benzo (a) pyrene (*)	1.5
2-Anthramine	0.6
Quinacrine HCl	0.6
Emodine	0.7
Nitrofluoren	0.7
2 Amino Biphenyl	25
9-10-Dimethyl-1.2-benzanthracen (*)	6.0
Aflatoxin-B_1 (*)	0.1
(3) DNA-Intercalating Agents	
Ethidium bromide	2.5
Acriflavin	0.1
9-Amino acridine	0.2
Proflavine-SO_4	0.2
Caffeine	20
Theophylline	20
Norharmane and Harmane	3
(4) DNA-Synthesis inhibitors and DNA damaging agents	
Mitomycin-C	0.5
Novobiocin	0.2
Nalidixic acid	5
Coumermycin	2
UV irradiation	100 erg/mm^2

The tested chemicals were dissolved in water or DMSO and their mutagenic activity was tested as described (24,26,28). Some agents (indicated by star) were tested in the presence of rat liver microsomes (S-9 preparation), in this system the rough mutant of Photobacterium leiognathi - 1827 was used . Levi and Ulitzur (in preparation) .

This phenotypical reversion of luminescence seems to be due to the un-repressed transcription of the luciferase cistron that resulted from the formation of a relaxation state of the DNA by the intercalating agents (26).

3) DNA synthesis inhibitors: This group includes DNA-damaging agents, such as mitomycin C or UV irradiation, as well as nalidixic acid and novobiocin (see Table 1). The present evidence supports the possibility that all of these agents act through their ability to trigger the "SOS functions" involved in the inactivation of the lumi-nescence system repressor (28).

The new Bioluminescence-Test is sensitive, rapid, very simple and cheap. Moreover it can be run automatically, using a scintillation counter, and the results are obtained within 12 hours. The Biolumi-nescence-Test appears to be, therefore an ideal short-term screening test to be employed in surveying suspected carcinogens. The positive responding chemicals should then be tested by a battery of in vitro tests, which will confirm or exclude their carcinogenicity potential. This approach may facilitate testing of more suspected chemicals, save money and allow a better use of the limited resources available for the comprehensive study of suspected carcinogens.

ACKNOWLEDGEMENTS

The author wishes to thank M. Barak, B. Levi and A. Naveh for providing data of their unpublished work.

REFERENCES

1. Chang, J.C., Taylor, P.B., and Franklin, R.L. (1981): Bull. Environm Contam. Toxicol. 26: 150-156.

2. Dalgneanlt R., Larouche, A., and Thibault, G. (1979): Clin. Chem. 25: 1639-1643.

3. Gorus, F. and Schram E. (1979): Clin. Chem. 25: 512-519.

4. Halsey, M.J. and Smith E.B.S. (1970): Nature, 227: 1363-1365.

5. Hastings, J.W. and Nealson, K.H. (1977): Annu. Rev. Microbiol., 31: 549-595.

6. Middleston, A.J. and Smith, E.B. (1976): Proc. R. Soc. Lond. B., 193:159-171.

7. Middleston, A.J., and Smith, E.D. (1976): Proc. R. Soc. Lond. B. 193: 173-190.

8. Nealson, K.H., and Hastings J.W. (1979): Microbiol. Rev. 43: 496-518.

9. Nilsson, L. (1978): Antimicrob. Agents Chemother., 14:812-816.

10. Oshino, R., Oshino, N., Tamura, M., Kobilinsky, L., and Chance, B. (1972): Biochim. Biophys. Acta. 273: 5-17.

11. Serat, W.F., Budinger Jr., F.E., and Kueller, P.K. (1967): Atmospheric Environment, Pergamon Press Vol. 1: 21-32.

12. Silva, M.T., Sousa, J.C.F., Polonia J.J., and Macedo, P.M. (1979): J. Bacteriol, 137: 461-468.

13. Thore A. (1979): Annals of Clinical Biochemistry, 16: 359-369.

14. Ulitzur, S., and Yashphe,J. (1975): Biochim. Biophys. Acta, 404: 321-328.

15. Ulitzur, S., and Heller M. (1978): Annal. Biochem., 91: 421-431.

16. Ulitzur, S. (1979): Biochem. Biophys. Acta, 572: 211-217.

17. Ulitzur, S. and Hastings, J.W. (1978): Methods in Enzymology Vol.57 189-193. Academic Press, New York.

18. Ulitzur, S. and Hastings, J.W. (1978): Proc. Natl. Acad. Sci. U.S.A. 75: 266-269.

19. Ulitzur, S., Yagen I., and Rottem, S. (1979): Env. and Appl. Bacteriol., 37: 782-784.

20. Ulitzur, S. and Hastings, J.W. (1979): Proc. Natl. Acad. Sci. U.S.A 76: 265-267.

21. Ulitzur, S., and Hastings, J.W. (1979): J. Bacteriol, 137: 854-859.

22. Ulitzur, S., and Hastings, J.W. (1979): Current Microbiol., 2: 345-348.

23. Ulitzur, S., and Heller, M. (1980): Methods in Enzymology, 72: 338-346. Academic Press, New York.

24. Ulitzur, S., Weiser, I., and Yannai, S. (1980): Mutat. Res., 74: 113-124.

25. Ulitzur, S., and Hastings, J.W. (1980): Current. Microbiol., 3: 295-300.

26. Ulitzur,S., and Weiser, I. (1981): Proc. Natl. Acad. Sci. U.S.A. (in press).

27. Varon, M., and Shilo, M. (1981): Microbial Ecology (in press)

28. Weiser, I., Ulitzur, S. and Yannai, S. (1981): Mutat. Res. (in press).

29. Whitehead, T.P., Kricka, L.J., Carter, T.J.N. and Thorpe, G.H.H., (1979): Clinical Chemistry, 25: 1531-1546.

Luminescent Assays: Perspectives in Endocrinology and Clinical Chemistry, edited by M. Serio and M. Pazzagli, Raven Press, New York © 1982.

Bioassay Procedures for Identifying Genotoxic Agents Using Light Emitting Bacteria as Indicator Organisms

Richard A. Wecher and *Stanley Scher

*Department of Biology and *School of Environmental Studies, Sonoma State University, Rohnert Park, California 94928*

Short-term microbial bioassays have been developed to identify environmental agents with the potential to cause damage to DNA (1). They provide a technically simple, rapid and inexpensive approach to detecting genotoxic properties of chemicals. The use of luminescent microorganisms as test objects for short-term bioassays is currently being investigated (3-5). Recent work has focussed on the determinants of light emission in the genus Photobacterium, a non-pathogenic member of the Enterobacteriaceae. Mutants have been isolated that exhibit rates of light emission that are several orders of magnitude lower than wild-type controls. When such mutants are exposed to sub-lethal concentrations of frameshift agents or base-substitution mutagens, light emission increases to near wild-type rates. Two methods of measurement have been employed: liquid-suspension assays using a scintillation counter to determine luminosity and plate incorporation assays to determine the frequency of bright clones in the treated population. We report here on the use of disc-diffusion assay procedures for identifying genotoxic properties of chemicals.

METHODS

Wild-type cells of Photobacterium phosphoreum were isolated as described previously (3). Mutant strains derived from P. phosphoreum showed rates of light emission that were 10^{-3} to 10^{-4} lower than controls.

Cells were grown as described previously (3). Absolute ethanol served as a solvent for chemicals poorly soluble in aqueous media. Acetone, benzene, chloroform, hydroxylamine, toluene and xylene were obtained from Mallinckrodt; caffeine, 1-naphthol and p-nitroanaline from Matheson C/B; ethyl carbamate was a gift from Dr. Ronald Baker; other chemicals were from Sigma.

For disc-diffusion assays, cells were grown in unshaken flasks at 23-25°C, diluted to 100-300 cells/0.1ml and spread on agar media. Sterile metricel discs of 0.6 cm diameter were aseptically placed near the center of the inoculated agar plate. Solutions of chemicals were applied to each disc in a volume of 0.1 ml. Plates were incubated for at least 18 hours at 23-25°C, and scored either visually after dark adaptation, or by photographing bright clones in total darkness. Bright clones were scored as those that were brighter than controls.

RESULTS AND DISCUSSION

For each compound listed in Table 1, we have reported the current carcinogenic status, and data indicating the response of the McCann et al (2) Salmonella microsome test (SAT) for comparison with P. phosphoreum strain (PPL⁻). In contrast to Salmonella and most other procaryotic microorganisms that have been employed as test objects for identifying genotoxic agents, Photobacteria do not appear to require an exogenous source of metabolic activating enzymes to convert promutagens into their active form(s). These results suggest that light-emitting microorganisms may possess one or more enzymes that are similar in function to the cytochrome P-450 mediated oxygenase system in mammalian microsomes.

The results presented here provide evidence that P. phosphoreum strain (PPL⁻) is responsive to a wide range of genotoxic agents. Acridines, acridinium and phenanthridium compounds known to cause frameshift mutations by intercalation markedly increase the frequency of bright clones. Similar results are obtained with aromatic solvents and other compounds for which animal studies suggest carcinogenic potential. When exposed to compounds such as hydroxylamine that are known to produce base pair transition by deamination of cytosine, the frequency of cells forming bright clones also increases.

Figure 1 shows the appearance of disc-diffusion assay plates containing decreasing concentrations of 3,6-diaminoacridine and appropriate controls. Mutagen induced bright clones appear as a ring around each disc. Thus the disc-diffusion assay provides a simple procedure for obtaining a preliminary estimate of genotoxic activity. The ability of light-emitting microorganisms to detect genotoxic properties of chemicals suggests that such assays may be useful for monitoring mutagenic compounds excreted in urine or present in other body fluids. In addition, when combined with chromatographic techniques, the light-emitting assay may be useful for identifying genotoxic components in complex environmental mixtures.

TABLE 1. Response of Salmonella typhimurium (SAT) microsome test and
         Photobacterium phosphoreum (PPL⁻) to potentially
         genotoxic compounds and appropriate controls.

Compound tested	Carcinogenic Status	SAT[a]	PPL⁻
3,6-bis (dimethylamino) acridine	+	+	+
3,6-diaminoacridine	b	+	+
3,6-diamino-10-methyl-acridinium chloride	b	e	+
3,8-diamino-5-ethyl-6-phenyl-phenanthridium bromide	c	+	+
chloroform	+	e	+
1-naphthol	b	o	+
1-naphthylamine	c	+	+
ethyl carbamate	+	o	+
caffeine	b	o	+
hydroxylamine	o	o	+
p-nitroanaline	b	e	+
xylene	d	e	+
toluene	d	e	+
benzene	c	o	+
ethyl alcohol	o	o	o
acetone	o	o	o
dimethylsulfoxide	o	o	o

a = S-9 fraction of rat liver induced with Arochlor 1254
b = status indefinite, inadequate data available
c = suspected carcinogen
d = carcinogenesis bioassay underway
e = not tested
+ = carcinogen/mutagen
o = non-carcinogen/non-mutagen

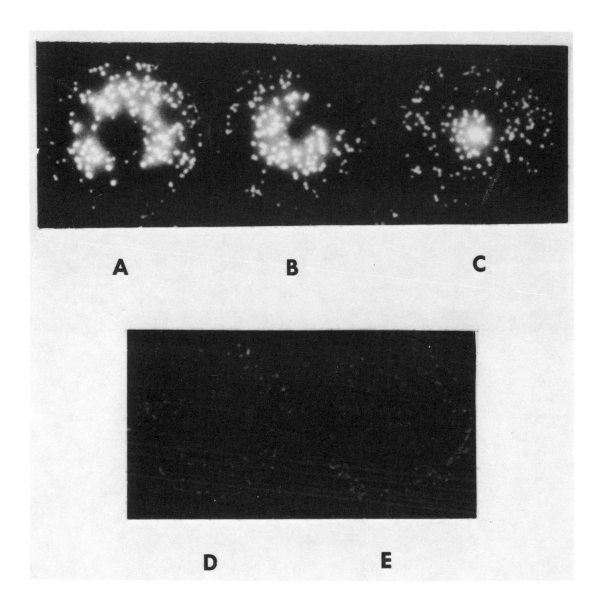

Figure 1. Disc-diffusion Assay.
   A. 3,6-diamino-acridine 100 ug/disc
   B. 3,6-diamino-acridine 10 ug/disc
   C. 3,6-diamino-acridine   1 ug/disc
   D. Ethanol 0.1 ml/disc
   E. Medium, unsupplemented 0.1 ml/disc

References:

1. Hollstein, M., McCann, J., Angelsanto, F.A. and Nichols, W.W. (1979). Short-term tests for carcinogens and mutagens. Mutation Research 65: 133-226.

2. McCann, J., Choi, E., Yamasaki, E. and Ames, B.N. (1975). Detection of carcinogens as mutagens in the Salmonella/microsome test: Assay of 300 chemicals. Proc. Nat. Acad. Sci. USA 72: 5135-5139.

3. Scher, S. and Wecher, R.A. (1981). Photon emitting micro-organisms as test objects for detecting genotoxic agents. In: Brookhaven National Laboratory Symposium on Genotoxic Effects of Airborne Agents. edited by R. Tice. (in press) Plenum Press, New York.

4. Ulitzur, S., Weiser, I. and Yannai, S. (1980). A new, sensitive and simple bioluminescence test for mutagenic compounds. Mutation Research 74: 113-124.

5. Ulitzur, S., Weiser, I. and Yannai, S. (1981). Bioluminescent test for mutagenic agents. In: Bioluminescence and Chemilumin-escence. edited by W. McElroy and M. deLuca. pp 139-145 Academic Press, New York.

Luminescent Assays: Perspectives in Endocrinology and Clinical Chemistry, edited by M. Serio and M. Pazzagli, Raven Press, New York © 1982.

Bioluminescent Assays of Clinically Important Compounds

Marlene DeLuca

Department of Chemistry, University of California at San Diego, La Jolla, California 92093

The use of bioluminescence for assaying many important biological molecules has been well documented. The advantage of bioluminescent assays is speed, sensitivity and specificity. The applications of the firefly luciferase have been discussed previously, so I will be presenting mainly applications of the bacterial system.

The luminescent bacteria *Beneckea harveyi* contain an NAD(P)H:FMN oxidoreductase and a luciferase which catalyze the following reactions.

$$(1)\ NAD(P)H + FMN + H^+ \xrightarrow{\text{oxidoreductase}} NAD(P)^+ + FMNH_2$$

$$(2)\ FMNH_2 + RCHO + O_2 \xrightarrow{\text{luciferase}} FMN + RCOOH + H_2O + h\nu$$

Reaction (1) is catalyzed by the oxidoreductase and the $FMNH_2$ produced can be utilized by luciferase in the presence of O_2 and a long chain aldehyde to produce light.

If the assay conditions are such that NAD(P)H is the limiting component, the light intensity is directly proportional to the concentration of NAD(P)H. Any reaction that leads to the production or disappearance of NAD(P)H can be measured using this system. Since many clinical assays are coupled to the appearance of NAD(P)H, this bioluminescent assay is of great potential importance.

RESULTS

Table 1 shows a representative list of compounds and enzymes we have assayed with the bacterial enzymes. There are many other examples in the literature which are too numerous to cite. For a comprehensive listing, see (6).

115

TABLE 1:   Substrates and Enzymes Assayed with the Bacterial
           Bioluminescent Assay

Compound	Levels of Detection	Reference
NADH	0.5-1000 pmoles	Ford-DeLuca, 1981
NADPH	0.5-1000 pmoles	Ford-DeLuca, 1981
Glucose-6-phosphate	2-100 pmoles	Jablonski-DeLuca, 1979
ETOH	0.003%-.012%	Haggerty, 1978
Testosterone	0.8 pmole-1000 pmoles	Ford-DeLuca, 1981
Androsterone	0.8 pmole-1000 pmoles	Ford-DeLuca, 1981
TNT	10 attomoles	Unpublished
Methotrexate	0.5-2 pmoles	Wannlund, et al., 1980
Lactate Dehydrogenase	0.001-1 pmole	Haggerty, et al., 1978
Alcohol Dehydrogenase	0.01-10 pmoles	Haggerty, et al., 1978
Glucose-6-P Dehydrogenase	0.001-1 pmole	Haggerty, et al., 1978
Hexokinase	0.001-1 pmole	Haggerty, et al., 1978

Originally most of these assays were developed using the soluble
oxidoreductase and luciferase and the appropriate coupling enzyme. We
discovered (4) that it was possible to immobilize these enzymes onto
glass and these immobilized enzymes were stable and reusable. Figure 1
shows a typical curve for increasing concentrations of alcohol dehydrogenase as assayed using the immobilized enzymes (3).

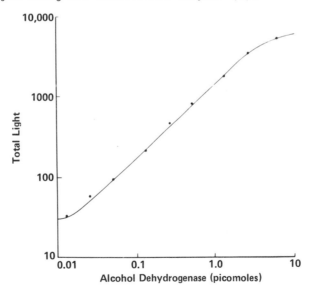

FIG. 1.   Determination of picomoles of alcohol dehydrogenase using immobilized luciferase and NADH:FMN oxidoreductase. Final concentrations of
the soluble components were 2×10^{-5} decanal, 2.3×10^{-6} M FMN, 3.4×10^{-1}
M ethanol, 9.4×10^{-3} M NAD, and soluble alcohol dehydrogenase in 0.1 M
potassium phosphate, pH 7.0.

Another advantage of the immobilized system is that for a given concentration of NADH in the range of 10-20 pmoles one obtains more light than with a comparable amount of soluble enzymes. These data are shown in Table 2. At very low concentrations of NADH, the immobilized and the soluble systems are comparable.

TABLE 2: Effect of NADH Concentration on Light Emission from Immobilized and Soluble Enzymes

NADH, pmole	Total Light	
	Immobilized	Soluble
2	500	823
5	2,330	2,170
10	7,260	4,810
20	31,680	10,950

We have recently found that immobilizing the enzymes on Sepharose rather than glass gives a product with much higher retention of enzymatic activity (2). We have examined the effects of co-immobilizing a third enzyme, glucose-6-phosphate dehydrogenase along with the oxidoreductase and luciferase.

Table 3 shows the data obtained when the enzymes are immobilized separately or together. Clearly the most efficient conversion of glucose-6-phosphate to light, in the coupled assay, is obtained when all three enzymes are immobilized simultaneously on the same Sepharose beads. At the highest concentration of glucose-6-phosphate there is about a 20-fold increase of light output from the co-immobilized enzymes relative to the separately immobilized enzymes. Similar observations have been reported for other co-immobilized multi-enzyme systems (7).

TABLE 3. Comparison of Light Obtained with Enzymes Co-immobilized or Separately Immobilized

Glucose-6-Phosphate pmoles	Light Intensity	
	Separately Immobilized	Co-Immobilized
20	0.9	2.6
200	2.0	25.6
2,000	16.0	240.0
20,000	119.0	2,400.0

We have also co-immobilized 3α or 3β, 17β hydroxysteroid dehydrogenase with the luminescent enzymes.

Figure 2 shows the light obtained as a function of androsterone or testosterone concentration. Light intensity was proportional to steroid concentration in the range of 0.5 pmoles to about 1 nmole. This assay is not quite as sensitive as an enzyme linked immunoassay (8), however, the immunoassay requires a 3-hour incubation while the bioluminescent assay is measured within 30 seconds. The bioluminescent assay is about 1000-fold more sensitive than a spectrophotometric method reported (1).

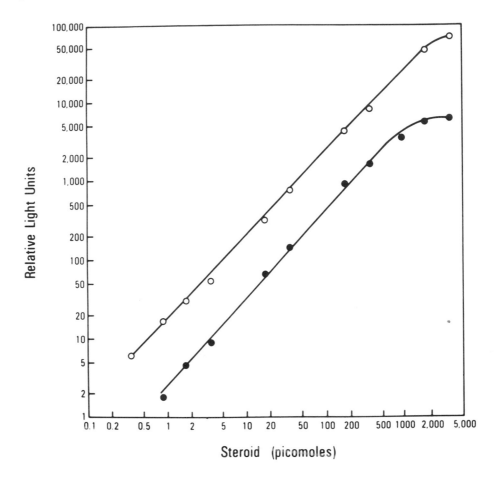

FIG. 2. Initial light intensity as a function of androsterone (o); or testosterone (•) concentration.

Immunoassays

Enzyme linked immunoassays have been used for some time. These assays generally utilize an enzyme with a high turnover number such as horseradish peroxidase or β galactosidase. We have developed a bioluminescent immunoassay for the methotrexate, utilizing firefly luciferase (9). The principle of this is illustrated in Fig. 3. Basically the antigen, methotrexate, is covalently linked to the luciferase and this conjugate is used in a competitive binding assay with varying concentrations of free antigens. We were able to obtain an enzyme-methotrexate conjugate containing approximately 2 moles of methotrexate per enzyme and retaining 70% of the catalytic activity.

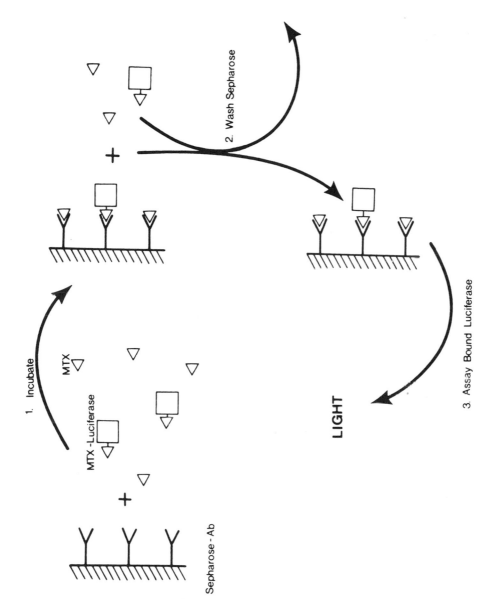

FIG. 3. Schematic representation of the steps in a bioluminescent immunoassay.

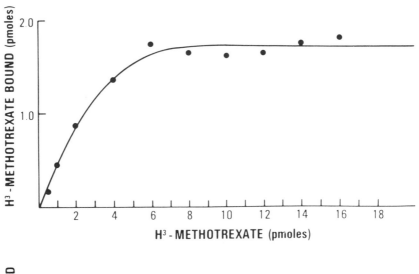

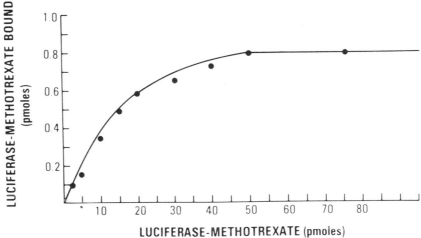

FIG. 4. Binding curves of ³H-methotrexate and luciferase-methotrexate
         to immobilized anti-methotrexate.

     We immobilized the antibody to Sepharose and compared the stoichio-
metry of binding of the conjugate with that of free methotrexate. This
is shown in Fig. 4. For a constant amount of antibody, 1.7 pmoles of
free methotrexate are bound and 0.8 pmoles of the methotrexate-lucifer-
ase are bound. So the methotrexate in the conjugate is available for
binding to the antibody. The rate of binding at 25°C is the same for
the free methotrexate or conjugate. They both exhibit maximal binding
within 1.5-2.0 hours.

A competitive binding curve is shown in Fig. 5. A constant amount of conjugate is incubated with the antibody in the presence of increasing amounts of free methotrexate. This assay is linear in the range of 0-10 pmoles of free methotrexate.

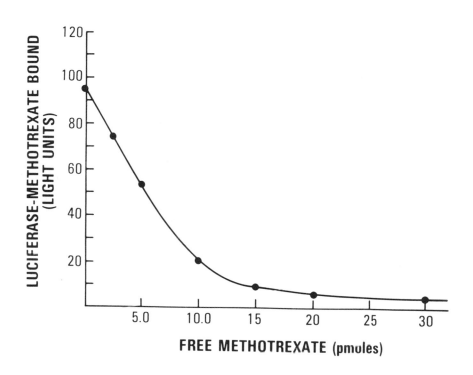

FIG. 5. Competitive binding curve of free methotrexate with luciferase-methotrexate to Sepharose antibody as measured by bioluminescence.

We also tried a double antibody technique where a rabbit antigoat IgG was used to precipitate the goat antibody-methotrexate complex. These results are shown in Figure 6. With this procedure as little as 50 femtomoles of methotrexate can be detected. It is our feeling that bioluminescent immunoassays can be developed for many other molecules of biological interest. Indeed with the appropriate amplification techniques we feel that detection in the attomole range is feasible.

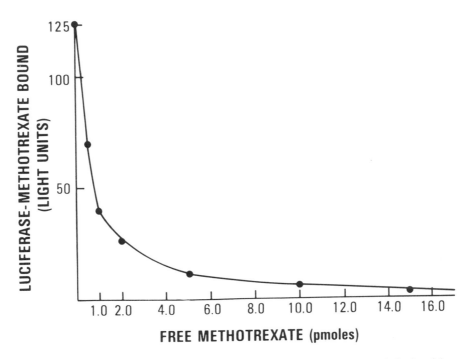

FIG. 6.   Competitive binding curve of free methotrexate with luciferase-
methotrexate using the double antibody technique.

ACKNOWLEDGEMENT

This work was supported by the National Institute of Health, Grant
GM 24621 and a contract from the United States Army (RFQ DAAK 70-79-A-
0019).

REFERENCES

1. Bovara, R., Carrea, G., Cremonesi, P., and Mazzola, G. (1981):
    Continuous-flow analysis of 3α hydroxysteroidd using immobilized
    3α-hydroxysteriod dehydrogenase. Anal. Biochem., 112: 239-243.
2. Ford, J., and DeLuca, M. (1981): A new assay for picomole levels
    of androsterone and testosterone using co-immobilized luciferase,
    oxidoreductase and steroid dehydrogenase. Anal. Biochem.,
    110: 43-48.
3. Haggerty, C., Jablonski, E., Stav, L., and DeLuca, M. (1978):
    Continuous monitoring of reactions that produce NADH and NADPH
    using immobilized luciferase and oxidoreductases from *Beneckea
    harveyi*. Anal. Biochem., 88: 162-173.
4. Jablonski, E., and DeLuca, M. (1976): Immobilization of bacterial
    luciferase and FMN reductase on glass rods. Proc. Natl. Acad. Sci.
    USA, 73: 3848-3851
5. Jablonski, E., and DeLuca, M. (1979): Properties and Uses of
    Immobilized Light Emitting Enzyme Systems for *Beneckea larveyi*.
    Clin. Chem., 25/9: 1622-1627.

6. Jablonski, E., and DeLuca, M.: In: <u>Clinical and Biochemical Applica-</u>
    <u>tions of Luminescence</u>, edited by L.J. Kricka, and T.J.N. Carter.
    Marcel-Dekker, New York. In press.
7. Mattiasson, B., and Mosbach, K., (1976): Multistep Enzyme Systems
    In: Methods in Enzymology, Vol. 44, edited by K. Mosbach, pp. 453-
    477. Academic Press, New York.
8. Rajkowski, K.M., Cittanova, N., Urios, P., and Jayle, M.F., (1977):
    Enzyme-Linked Immunoassay of Testosterone. Steroids, <u>30</u>, 129.
9. Wannlund, J., Azari, J., Levine, L., and DeLuca, M., (1980): A
    bioluminescent immunoassay for methotrexate at the sub-picomole
    level. <u>Biochem. Biophys. Res. Comm.</u>, <u>96</u>, pp. 440-446.

Luminescent Assays: Perspectives in Endocrinology and Clinical Chemistry, edited by M. Serio and M. Pazzagli, Raven Press, New York © 1982.

Bioluminescent Immunoassays: A Model System for Detection of Compounds at the Attomole Level

J. Wannlund, *H. Egghart, and M. DeLuca

*Chemistry Department, University of California, La Jolla, California 92093; *Mobility Equipment Research and Development Command, Fort Belvoir, Virginia 22060*

Numerous clinically important compounds are currently determined by radioimmunoassays (1). To void the inconvenience and stability problems associated with radiolabels, we have developed a bioluminescent immunoassay (BIA) for the detection of TNT. The detection of TNT is used as a model system to illustrate the feasibility of low level detection using bioluminescence. Bioluminescent immunoassay's exhibit greater specificity over chemiluminescent immunoassays in the presence of oxidizing species, because the luciferase will only emit light in the presence of its substrate.

We have developed two techniques for detecting compounds using bioluminescent immunoassays. The first is a direct labeling of the luciferase with the antigen (standard BIA) and the second is the labeling of an amplifying enzyme with the antigen (amplified BIA). The first system detects TNT at the femtomolar (10^{-15} moles) range and the amplified technique detects TNT to the attomolar range (10^{-18} moles).

Standard Bioluminescent Immunmoassays

Trinitrobenzene sulfonic acid (TNBS) is reacted with firefly luciferase to produce a TNP luciferase conjugate in a ratio of one mole of Trinitrophenyl (TNP) per mole of luciferase. The modified luciferase retains 80% of its catalytic activity. The antibody to TNT is covalently attached to Sepharose for easier handling and washing of unbound antigen. The procedure for this system is illustrated in Figure 1. The number of binding sites on the Sepharose antibody for both ^{3}H-TNT and TNP-luciferase were determined and found to be the same. So it appears that all of the antibody binding sites are available to the free antigen and the TNP-luciferase conjugate. A competitive binding curve with increasing amounts of free TNT is shown in Figure 2. The lower detection limit of TNT is at 50 femtomoles (5×10^{-14} moles). Similar results for the detection of dinitrophenol (DNP) using this same technique have been reported by Wannlund, et al, (2).

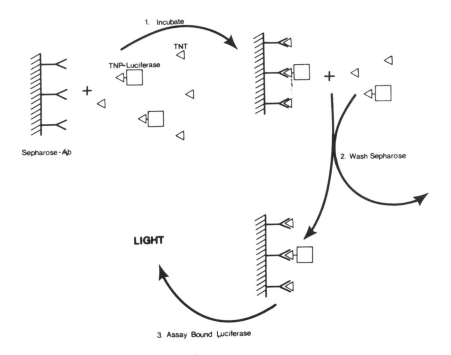

FIG. 1. The Procedure for a Bioluminescent Immunoassay: (1) Free antigen and luciferase-antigen are incubated with Sepharose-antibody; (2) Unbound antigen and luciferase-antigen are removed by washing; (3) The amount of bound luciferase-antigen is measured by light production.

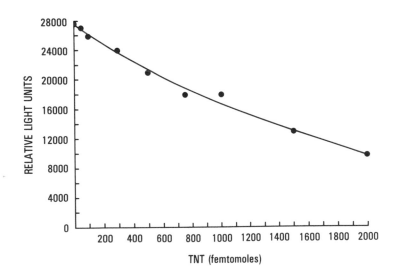

Fig. 2. The competitive binding of luciferase-TNP conjugate to Sepharose-anti-TNT with increasing amounts of free trinitrotoluene (TNT).

Amplified Bioluminescent Immunoassay Technique

This amplified technique uses a glucose-6-phosphate dehdyrogenase-Trinitrophenyl (G-6-PDH-TNP) conjugate instead of a luciferase-TNP conjugate for the detection of TNT. This enzyme was chosen because it has a large turnover number (70,000) and because it continually produces a molecule, NADH, which can be detected at low levels by the bacterial oxidoreductase and luciferase enzymes. Glucose-6-phosphate dehydrogenase catalyzes the reaction of glucose-6-phosphate (G-6-P) + $NAD^+ \rightleftharpoons$ glucono-δ-lactone-6-phosphate + NADH + H^+. The glucose-6-phosphate dehydrogenase enzyme has a specific activity of about 400 IU/mg. Thus one attomole (10^{-18} moles) of glucose-6-phosphate dehydrogenaase will generate 40 femtomoles of NAD/min.

TNBS is reacted with glucose-6-phosphate dehydrogenase to produce a glucose-6-phosphate dehydrogenase-TNP conjugate in a ratio of one mole of TNP per mole of glucose-6-phosphate dehydrogenase. The modified glucose-6-phosphate dehydrogenase retains 90% of its catalytic activity. The procedure used for the amplified bioluminescent immunoassay technique is illustrated in Figure 3. Both ^{3}H-TNT and glucose-6-phosphate dehydrogenase-TNP were used

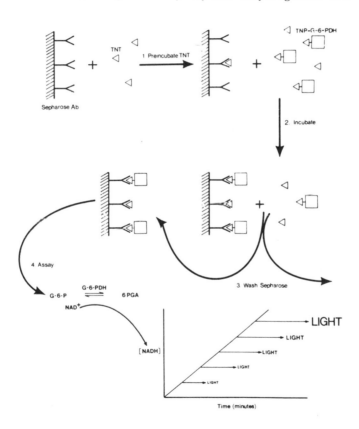

FIG. 3.   The procedure is essentially the same as in Fig. 1 except the antigen is bound to glucose-6-phosphate dehydrogenase (G-6-PDH).   Glucose-6-phosphate dehydrogenase-antigen bound to the Sepharose-Ab is allowed to react with glucose-6-phosphate (G-6-P) and NAD for 10 minutes and the resulting NADH is measured with the bacterial oxidoreductase-luciferase enzyme system.

to determine the number of binding sites on the Sepharose antibody.   Both resulted with the same number of binding sites on the Sepharose antibody. Therefore the binding sites are equally accessible to both the free TNT and the glucose-6-phosphate dehydrogenase-TNP conjugate.   The light measured when increasing amounts of free TNT are added is shown in Figure 4.   The lower detectable limit of TNT is 10 attomoles (10^{-17} moles).

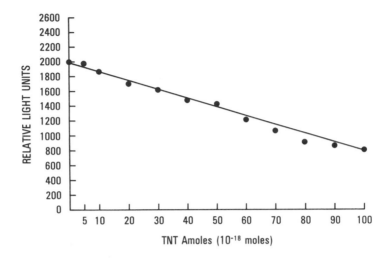

FIG. 4. The binding of glucose-6-phosphate dehydrogenase-TNP (G-6-PDH-TNP) to Sepharose-anti-TNT with increasing amounts of free TNT as measured with the bacterial oxidoreductase and luciferase enzyme system.

DISCUSSION

The lower limit of detection of TNT does not represent the theoretical limit of detection for this system. Further development of various parameters of the system including the use of higher affinity antibody and the improvement of assay procedures will increase the sensitivity of antigen detection.   This dynamic new technique using bioluminescence is adaptable for the ultrasensitive detection of virtually any compound to be measured.

ACKNOWLEDGEMENT

This work was supported by a contract from the United States Army (DAAK70-79-C-0174).

REFERENCES

1.   Travis, J. (1980): Clinical Radioimmunoassay ...State-of-the-Art, Radioassay Ligand Assay Publishers, Anaheim.
2.   Wannlund, J. and DeLuca, M. (1981): Bioluminescent Immunoassays: Use of Luciferase-Antigen Conjugates for Determination of Methotrexate and DNP. In: Bioluminescence and Chemiluminescence: Basic Chemistry and Analytical Applications, edited by M. DeLuca and W. McElroy, pp. 693-696. Academic Press, New York.

Luminescent Assays: Perspectives in Endocrinology and Clinical Chemistry, edited by M. Serio and M. Pazzagli, Raven Press, New York © 1982.

Luminescent Immunoassays and Binding Assays Monitored by Chemilumigenic Labels

Hartmut R. Schroeder

Ames Research and Development Laboratory, Miles Laboratories, Inc., Elkhart, Indianapolis 46515

Many substances of clinical interest are present at low levels in complex body fluids and are commonly measured by protein-binding radioassays. In these methods the ligand and a radiolabeled analog of the ligand compete for a limited number of binding sites, such as those on an antibody. The amount of free or bound radiolabeled ligand is related to the concentration of unlabeled ligand by means of standards.

Several modifications of the competitive binding (CPB) radio-assay are employed. For instance, in a two-site immunoradiometric procedure, an antigen contained in the sample is allowed to react with a specific antibody immobilized on a solid phase. After an incubation period and wash steps, excess radiolabeled antibody is added to detect the antigen. During a second incubation the antigen becomes sandwiched between the solid phase and radiolabeled antibodies (sandwich assay). Free radiolabeled antibody is removed by washing and the bound radiolabel is measured. Since reagents can be used in excess, this assay possesses great sensitivity and is useful for detection of high-molecular weight antigens.

The inconvenience of licensing and safety, as well as stability problems with radiolabels make non-radioisotopic labels desirable. Consequently, radiolabels have been replaced by enzymes (8,16,20), substrates (1), cofactors (9,2) and fluorescent dyes (18). In addition, chemilumigenic compounds have been used as highly sensitive labels, which are detected in a few seconds in simple light generating oxidation reactions (10,14,19). In this paper, I will describe our experiences using chemilumigenic labels to monitor both homogeneous and heterogeneous protein binding assays.

ASSAY PRINCIPLE

Heterogeneous immunoassay employing chemilumigenic labels follow procedures similar to those of radioassays. The ligand

129

of interest is covalently coupled to a chemilumigenic compound,
such as isoluminol, through standard amide bond-forming reactions.
The chemilumigenic conjugate then substitutes for the radiolabeled
ligand in a radioassay procedure. After completion of the immunoassay the amount of conjugate in the isolated bound fraction is
determined in a detection reaction. A catalyst, such as microperoxidase, and an oxidizing agent, such as hydrogen peroxide, are added
to produce light, which is proportional to the concentration of the
conjugate.

Homogeneous assays monitored by chemilumigenic labels eliminate
the separation step, but are otherwise similar to the heterogeneous
assays. Because the chemiluminescence efficiency of bound and free
forms of the labeled ligand can differ markedly, it is possible to
measure one in the presence of the other.

DETECTION OF CHEMILUMIGENIC LABELS

The detection limits for chemilumigenic compounds depend on
the efficiency of light production which is based on the structure
of the compounds and the reaction conditions (11,12). The amino-
phthalhydrazides, luminol (5-amino-2,3-dihydrophthalazine-1,4-dione)
and isoluminol (6-amino-2,3-dihydrophthalazine-1,4-dione, are
efficient light producers. We chose isoluminol for the label
although it produces less light than luminol. Alkylation of the
primary amino group at the 6 position increases light production,
while similar substitution at the 5 position decreases the
efficiency. The amino group of isoluminol was derivatized with an
amino alkyl side chain to allow coupling to ligands of interest
through stable amide bonds. Further alkylation of the 6-amino group
provided a label nearly as efficient in light production as luminol.
Although the chemical nature of the bridging arm had little effect
on chemiluminescence, intramolecular quenching was observed with some
ligands. Other chemilumigenic substances, such as the aminonaphthal-
hydrazides, can be detected at lower levels (0.1 pM) than the
isoluminol derivatives (1 pM), but they are poorly soluble at pH < 10.

Among numerous detection reactions for the above labels, heme
catalyzed oxidation with hydrogen peroxide is the most sensitive (11).
N,N-Diethylisoluminol and luminol were detectable at 1 pM concentration with a peak light intensity (PLI) or total light production of
1.5 times the background signal.

The hydrogen peroxide-microperoxidase oxidation systems were
unique in allowing equally sensitive reactions at pH 8.6 to 13.
Above pH 9.7, light emission from diethylisoluminol reached a peak
in about 0.70 sec. and decayed with a halflife of 4.5 seconds.
However, at pH less than 9.4 the kinetics were more rapid and the peak
light intensity was attained by about 0.22 sec. and decayed with a half
life of 0.5 seconds. The peak light intensities obtained in borate,
barbital or phosphate buffer at pH 8.6 were equivalent, but those in
Tris-HCl were only about one-third as great. Furthermore, small
amounts of protein in the system at pH 13, e.g. 0.1% serum, reduced
the peak light intensity by 50% over reactions without proteins, but
had little effect at this level in similar reactions at pH 8.6.

Chemiluminescence measurements have been plagued with large variability. Addition of hydrogen peroxide from a syringe with a Teflon-tipped plunger eliminates the variability caused by contact with metal. Thus, the PLI produced by N,N-diethylisoluminol in the presence of microperoxide at pH 13 had a coefficient of variation of only ±2% for the mean value of five reactions in triplicate (11). An experimental flow system reduced the coefficient of variation for six individual measurements to only 2.3%, without loss in sensitivity (13). This suggests that chemiluminescence measurements can be made much more reproducible.

A HOMOGENEOUS COMPETITIVE PROTEIN BINDING ASSAY FOR BIOTIN

The first demonstration of the potential usefulness of chemilumigenic labels to monitor protein binding reactions is illustrated in the following homogeneous assay for biotin (10).

Materials and Methods

Biotinyl-isoluminol Conjugate: Isoluminol was coupled to the carboxyl group of biotin via an aminohydroxypropyl bridging arm (10) to produce 6-(3-biotinylamido-2-hydroxypropylamino-2,3-dihydrophthalazine-1,4-dione, shown in Fig. 1.

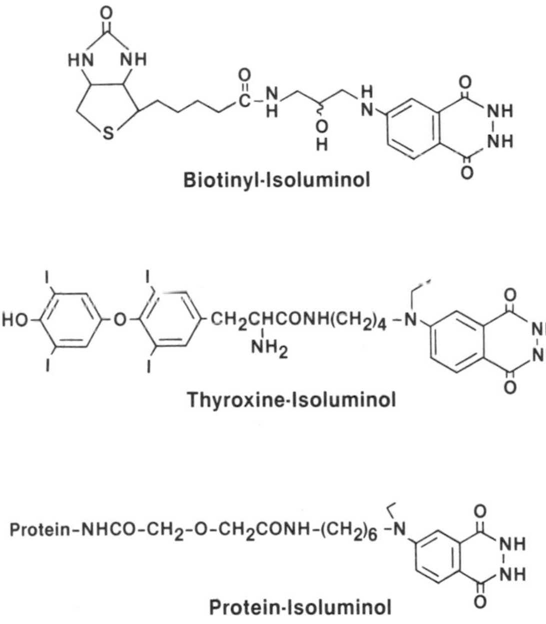

Biotinyl-Isoluminol

Thyroxine-Isoluminol

Protein-Isoluminol

FIG. 1 Structures of chemilumigenic conjugates.

Avidin: A stock solution of lyophilized avidin (Sigma Chemical Co., St. Louis, MO) at 1 mg/mL was made in 10 mM Tris-HCl, pH 7.4.

Lactoperoxidase: A stock solution of this enzyme (Calbiochem, San Diego, CA) was prepared in 0.1 M Tris-HCl, pH 7.4.

Light Measurements: A DuPont 760 Luminescence Biometer was used
to measure light produced in 6 x 50 mm tubes containing 150 μL of the
chemilumigenic compound and a catalyst. Chemiluminescence was initiated by addition of 10 μL of oxidant from a 25 μL Hamilton syringe.
The PLI's were measured directly and total light production was monitored with a recorder.

H_2O_2-Lactoperoxidase Oxidation System: A 10 μL aliquot of 0.95 mM
H_2O_2 was added to the chemilumigenic compound and 10 μg of lactoperoxidase in 150 μL of 0.1 M Tris-HCl, pH 7.4.

Titration of Avidin With Biotinyl-Isoluminol: Reaction mixtures
(140 μL) containing 84 nM biotinyl-isoluminol and various levels of
avidin in 0.1 M Tris-HCl, pH 7.4, were incubated at 25°C for 15 min.
Then 10 μL of lactoperoxidase (10 μg) and 10 μL of H_2O_2 were added to
produce light. The PLIs from binding reactions performed in triplicate
were averaged.

Biotin Assay: Binding reactions (140 μL) were assembled with biotin at various concentrations, 90 nM biotin-isoluminol and 3.7 μg
avidin/mL (added last) in 0.1 M Tris-HCl, pH 7.4. After 5 min incubation at 25°C, reactions were monitored with the H_2O_2-lactoperoxidase
system as above.

RESULTS

An interesting model assay for biotin was developed with biotinyl-
isoluminol. On oxidation in the H_2O_2-lactoperoxidase system biotinyl-
isoluminol produced about one-half as much light as the isoluminol label
and was detectable at levels as low as 5 nM. An unusual phenomenon
occurred when a constant amount of biotinyl-isoluminol was first incubated with increasing levels of avidin, the natural binding protein
for biotin, and then oxidized. The PLI, as well as the total light
production, increased ten-fold as the avidin concentration rose to
14 μg/mL (Fig. 2). Greater levels of avidin reduced the enhancement
in chemiluminescence due to a general protein effect. Since the PLI
produced with the isoluminol derivative label was unchanged by pre-
incubation with avidin, the enhancement was specific.

The increased chemiluminescence efficiency of biotinyl-isoluminol
when complexed by avidin permitted assembly of a homogeneous CPB assay.
Biotin at various concentrations was allowed to compete with a constant
amount of biotinyl-isoluminol for a limited number of avidin binding
sites. The PLI produced with these binding reaction mixtures on oxidation with H_2O_2 and lactoperoxidase decreased as the level of biotin
increased (Fig. 3). The lower detection limit with this partially
optimized assay was 50 nM biotin.

This work illustrated that a homogeneous CPB assay could be
monitored with a chemilumigenic label. The assay was simplified
because the enhanced light yield of the biotinyl-isoluminol-avidin
complex over that of the conjugate itself eliminated the need for a
separation step. However, this format limits sensitivity since free
biotinyl-isoluminol, also present in the reaction mixture, contributes
a substantial background signal.

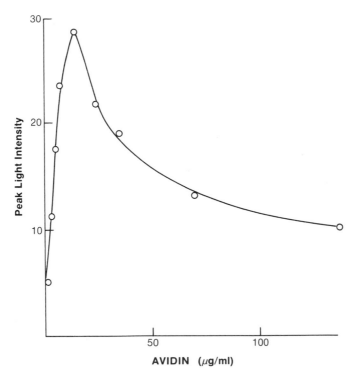

FIG. 2   Effect of avidin on PLI produced with biotinyl-isoluminol.

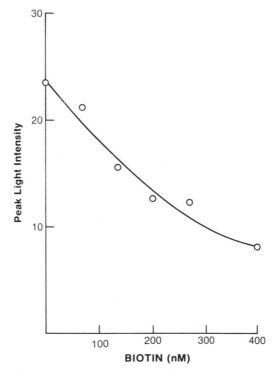

FIG. 3.   Homogeneous CPB assay for biotin.   Reproduced as in Fig. 2.

The above approach was briefly considered for determination of thyroxine (T_4) in serum. Although the light yield of a chemilumigenic T_4 conjugate increased after complexing by its antibody binding partner, the maximum enhancement was only 2.5-fold (12). Furthermore, serum components other than T_4, such as proteins, quenched chemiluminescence significantly (12). This additional limitation of a homogeneous method made a heterogeneous procedure more desirable. Nevertheless, a homogeneous chemiluminescence immunoassay (CIA) for progesterone in serum was practical because a pre-extraction step with organic solvents eliminated interference problems and was also required by the radioimmunoassay (RIA) (4). The CIA determined as little as 25 pg of progesterone and compared favorably to the RIA.

HETEROGENEOUS IMMUNOASSAY FOR SERUM THYROXINE

The following description of a heterogeneous CIA for thyroxine (T_4) in serum indicates the utility of chemilumigenic labels for monitoring clinical samples (14).

Materials and Methods

Thyroxine-Isoluminol: A more efficient isoluminol derivative was coupled to the carboxyl group of thyroxine by means of mixed anhydride to produce 6-[N-ethyl-N-(4-thyroxinylamido-n-butylamino)]-2,3-dihydrophthalazine-1,4-dione, shown in Fig. 1. Stock solutions of 1 mM T_4-isoluminol in 0.1 M Na_2CO_3, pH 9.5, were kept at 4° and diluted in 0.1 M NaOH just before use.

Thyroxine: Working standards of T_4 (Sigma Chemical Corp., St. Louis, MO) were prepared in 10% serum (striped of T_4 with charcoal) in 0.1 M NaOH.

Antibody to Thyroxine: Antibody to a T_4-bovine serum albumin conjugate was raised in rabbits and isolated by ammonium sulfate precipitation of the antiserum.

Microperoxidase: A stock solution of microperoxidase (Sigma Chemical Corp.) at 0.4 mg/mL (0.2 mM) in 10 mM Tris-HCl, pH 7.4 was stable at 4° for at least one month. Dilutions to 2 µM were made in 75 mM barbital (N,N-diethylbarbiturate) buffer, pH 8.6, just prior to use.

Light Measurement: Chemiluminescence was determined on the Biometer as before, except that the H_2O_2 was added from a custom-built automatic injection device (14).

H_2O_2 - Microperoxidase Oxidation System at pH 12.6: A catalyst solution consisting of 20 µL of 2 µM microperoxidase in barbital buffer and 35 µL of 0.2 M NaOH was mixed with the chemilumigenic compound in 95 µL of 75 mM barbital buffer (final pH 12.6). After a ten min incubation, a 10 µL aliquot of 90 mM H_2O_2 in 10 mM Tris-HCl, pH 7.4, was injected. The PLI was measured and averaged for reactions performed in triplicate.

Thyroxine Assay: Five picomoles of T_4-isoluminol in 200 µL of 0.1 M NaOH were applied to columns packed with 1 mL of Sephadex G-25

and washed into the bed with 1 mL of 0.1 N NaOH. Then standard solutions of T_4 (200 μL) or serum samples diluted 1:10 in 0.1 N NaOH
(200 μL) were added. The columns were washed with 4 mL of 75 mM
barbital, pH 8.6, to remove interfering serum components. The CPB
reaction was initiated with addition of 0.3 mL of antibody to T_4
(sufficient to bind 60% of the T_4-isoluminol in the absence of
competing T_4). After 1 h incubation, the antibody was eluted with
0.8 mL of barbital buffer. Antibody bound T_4-isoluminol was determined from the PLI produced by 95 μL aliquots of the eluate in the
H_2O_2-microperoxidase system, pH 12.6. CPB reactions were performed
in triplicate and PLI values were averaged.

Results

We evaluated an immunoassay for serum thyroxine that was monitored with the chemilumigenic T_4 conjugate. The light yield of T_4-
isoluminol in the H_2O_2-microperoxidase system was only 2% as much as
the label itself. This loss in quantum efficiency was caused by
intramolecular quenching from the rather bulky iodine atoms on the
T_4 portion of the molecule. Nonetheless, T_4-isoluminol was detectable
to a lower limit of 0.1 nM, which was adequate for the CIA.
Competitive protein binding reactions were carried out on columns
containing Sephadex G-25, which binds both T_4 and T_4-isoluminol. For
effective competition both thyroxine species should occupy the same
column volume element. However, since T_4-isoluminol migrated more
slowly than T_4, the conjugate was applied first and washed part way
into the gel bed with 0.1 N NaOH. Then, the serum sample was diluted
in 0.1 N NaOH and added for quantitative extraction of T_4. Serum
components other than thyroxine were washed from the column with
barbital buffer, pH 8.6. This step eliminated interference problems
in the binding reaction and subsequent chemiluminescence detection
reaction. Antibody at appropriate dilution was applied to the column
and a 1-h incubation followed. The antibody-bound T_4 was eluted with
buffer and determined from the PLI produced with aliquots of the
effluent in the H_2O_2-microperoxidase system.

A standard curve was generated for relating PLI to T_4 concentration (Fig. 4). Increasing concentrations of T_4 diminished the
amount of T_4-isoluminol bound to antibody, and consequently lowered
the PLI obtained with this fraction. The CIA was useful for determining T_4 levels in the clinically significant range of 25-200 nM.
The specificity of the assay was confirmed when isoluminol substituted
for the conjugate produced no response. Results obtained with 28
serums correlated reasonably well with those of the Tetralute RIA
(Ames Co., Miles Laboratories, Elkhart, IN 46515) as reference (Fig. 5).
The reproducibility and assay time of the CIA were similar to those
of the RIA. Although less convenient for routine use than the RIA,
this example demonstrated the feasibility of monitoring immunoassays
with chemilumigenic labels.

SOLID PHASE IMMUNOASSAYS FOR HEPATITIS B SURFACE ANTIGEN
IN SERUM AND ANTI-HUMAN IgG

Recently we developed a double-antibody, sandwich immunoassay for
detection of hepatitis B surface antigen (HB_sAg) by means of a chemilum-

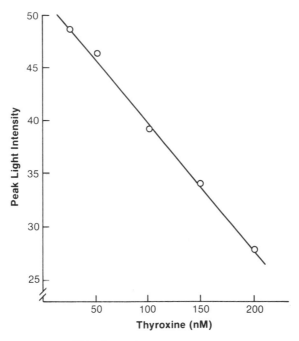

FIG. 4 Heterogeneous CIA for thyroxine in serum. Reproduced by permission, Elsevier/North Holland Biomedical Press.

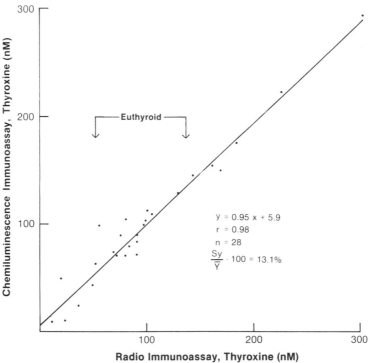

FIG. 5 Comparison of CIA and RIA methods for determination of thyroxine levels in clinical sera. Reproduced as in Fig. 4.

igenic label in order to determine the sensitivity of this approach for large molecular weight ligands (15).

Materials and Methods

Anti-HB Ag: Rabbits were injected with HB_s Ag purified by $CsCl_2$ density-gradient centrifugation. Anti-HB_s Ag was isolated from the antiserum by chromatography on DE-52 ion-exchange cellulose. Highly purified anti-HB_s Ag was obtained by immunoprecipitation and density gradient centrifugation at low pH (5).

Preparation of Protein-Isoluminol Conjugates: A isoluminol derivative with a carboxyalkyl bridging arm, 6-[carboxymethoxy-acetyl-N-(6-aminohexyl)-N-ethylamino]-2,3-dihydrophthalazine-1,4-dione (or CM-AHEI) was coupled to protein amino groups by a two-step procedure. First, 20 μmole of CM-AHEI and 20 μmole of N-hydroxysuccinimide were dissolved in 204 μL of dry N,N-dimethylformamide (DMF) under nitrogen. The solution was cooled to -10°C combined with 23 μmole of N,N-dicyclo-hexylcarbodiimide in 46 μL of DMF and incubated overnight at 0°C. Then, 5 μL of the active ester was rapidly mixed with 1 mg of either highly purified anti-HB_s Ag or human IgG (Pentex, Fraction II, Miles Laboratories, Inc., Elkhart, IN) in 1 mL of 0.1 M sodium phosphate - 0.15 M NaCl, pH 8.0. After 2.5 h at 4°C and 0.5 h at 20°C, the labeled conjugate product was solubilized with Tween 20 at 0.25%. The mixture was applied to a 1.5 x 48 cm column packed with Sephadex G-25 and eluted with 25 mM Tris-HCl-250 mM NaCl, pH 8.6. The isolated chemilumigenic anti-HB_s Ag conjugate (Fig. 1) was stabilized with normal human and normal rabbit serum at 15% (v/v) each, azide at 0.1% and storage at 4°C.

The number of AHEI labels covalently attached to protein was estimated from the absorbance of the conjugate at 325 nM (AHEI ε 12500 $M^{-1} cm^{-1}$). Active labels incorporated were determined from the light yield of the conjugate compared to that of AHEI in the H_2O_2-microperoxidase system at pH 12.6 as described earlier. Protein was precipitated with trichloroacetic acid at 10%, centrifuged and analyzed by Lowry assay using bovine serum albumin as standard (6).

Light Measurements: A computer-directed luminometer was developed in-house for automated readout of immunoassays performed in microtiter plates made of polyvinyl chloride (#1-220-29, Dynatec Laboratories, Alexandria, VA). The wells were covered with plastic tape and the plate was placed in the carrier which positioned individual wells over a phototube (Fig. 6). Pneumatically driven needles pierced the tape cover and added 100 μL of microperoxidase, followed 5 sec later by 20 μL of H_2O_2, from pressurized vessels. The light produced was measured for two seconds by photon counting (EMI-9789A, low noise, housing amplifier 3262/Ad, PMT with discriminator 3/N 323 from Pacific Precision Instruments, Concord, CA) and displayed by a printer.

H_2O_2-Microperoxidase System at pH 8.6: The luminometer added 100 μL of 2 μM microperoxidase in 50 mM borate, pH 8.6, to wells containing a protein sandwich completed with a chemilumigenic conjugate. After 5 sec 20 μL of 5 mM H_2O_2 in 10 mM Tris-HCl, pH 7.4 were injected and photons emitted were counted.

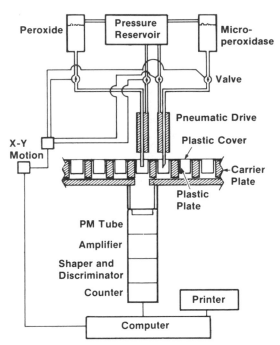

FIG. 6 Schematic of the luminometer. Reproduced by permission,
Clinical Chemistry

Solid Phase Anti-HB Ag: Each well of a microtiter plate was
incubated with 100 µL of partially purified anti-HB$_s$Ag at 25 µg/mL
($\varepsilon_{1\%}^{1 \ cm}$ 11.7 at 280 nm) in 0.1 M Na$_2$CO$_3$ - 0.1% NaN$_3$, pH 9.5. Plates
were sealed with SARAN® wrap and stored at 4° for 1 to 30 days. Just
prior to use the plates were washed three times with 180 µL per well
of 10 mM phosphate-140 mM NaCl, pH 7 (PBS) on a miniwash apparatus
(Model B, #2-315, Dynatec).

Solid Phase Human IgG: Wells were coated with 100 µL of human
IgG at 0.5 µg/mL for 6 h at 20°C, followed with bovine serum albumin
(BSA) at 1 mg/mL overnight at 4°C.

CIA for HB Ag: Serum samples (100 µL) or HB$_s$Ag positive reference
sera diluted in normal human serum were added to individual wells of the
anti-HB$_s$Ag coated plates. After 2-h incubation at 40°C, the plates were
washed (miniwash apparatus) three times with 180 µL of PBS per well.
Then 100 µL of chemilumigenic anti-HB$_s$Ag conjugate at 0.13 µg/mL in 15%
BSA (PENTEX®, 30% solution, Miles Laboratories, Inc., Elkhart, IN) - PBS
was added to 12 wells at a time with a multichannel pipette (Flow Laboratories, Inc., McLean, VA) and a second 2-h incubation at 40°C followed.
The plates were washed six times with PBS, covered with tape and placed
in the luminometer for automatic readout of chemiluminescence. For
dose-response curves, the photon count from six replicates was averaged.
Serums were analyzed singly. Since the photon count contained a constant chemical background, the lower detection limit was defined as
the mean count plus four standard deviations obtained with eight
replicate negative controls run on each plate.

A confirmation test with HB$_s$Ag positive sera was conducted by neutralizing the antigen after the first incubation (above) with 100 µL of human anti-HB$_s$Ag per well for 30 min at 40° and completing the assay as above.

CIA for Anti-Human IgG: Contrived samples consisting of various amounts of rabbits anti-human IgG (Cappel Laboratories, Inc., Cochranville, PA) in 100 µL of 1% BSA-PBS were added to the human IgG coated wells of a microtiter plate. After 1.5 h at 40°C plates were washed three times with PBS. Then the sandwich was completed by addition of 100 µL of chemilumigenic human IgG at 0.26 µg/mL in 15% BSA-PBS and incubation for 1.5 h at 40°C. The final wash and readout were as above.

RESULTS

A sandwich CIA for HB$_s$Ag was developed which employed a highly efficient chemilumigenic isoluminol derivative as label. Previous heterogeneous CIAs for proteins utilized luminol coupled to IgG via Schiffs base (3) and diazotization (17). However, these conjugates retained only 20 and 0.7% of the quantum efficiency of luminol, respectively. We selected active ester chemistry for coupling because this approach avoids unwanted side reactions of bifunctional coupling agents. An aminoalkylisoluminol derivative, AHEI, was reacted with diglycolic anhydride (15) to introduce a carboxy group. It was converted to the N-hydroxysuccinimide ester under anhydrous conditions and then reacted with aqueous protein at pH 8 to form the desired conjugate (Fig. 1). Labeling was first optimized with human IgG and then corroberated with the highly purified anti-HB$_s$Ag which was in short supply. Consequently, a CIA for anti-human IgG was also developed to evaluate chemilumigenic human IgG conjugates.

Conditions for coupling of CM-AHEI to human IgG were investigated systematically. Conjugates were evaluated on the basis of incorporation of label and performance in the CIA. A high active ester to IgG ratio (Fig. 7) and high pH favored incorporation. However, the incorporation estimated from chemiluminescence yield was lower than that estimated from absorbance measurements. The difference was greatest at low label to IgG ratios, high pH and high temperature (some data not shown). This loss in chemilumigenic activity of the label may be caused by self-polymerization of CM-AHEI, coupling through the heterocyclic ring portion, and intra-molecular quenching by protein (15). CIAs were conducted with each conjugate at 0.25 µg/mL concentration. The slopes of the initial linear portion of the resulting dose-response curves were maximal with conjugates produced at intermediary levels of active ester label per mg IgG (Fig. 7). Meanwhile the non-specific binding was nearly constant, but rose drastically with the conjugate bearing 31 labels. Thus, highly labeled conjugates gave less sensitive CIAs despite better agreement in incorporation estimates because of loss in immunoreactivity and greater non-specific binding. Under the best conditions (Materials and Methods) with 5 µL of active ester per mg, both human IgG and anti-HB$_s$Ag incorporated about seven AHEI by spectral and 0.5 by chemiluminescence estimate (molar ratio, Fig. 7). The immunoreactivity of this anti-HB$_s$Ag after labeling was unchanged according to the AUSAB® test (Abbott Laboratories, N. Chicago, IL).

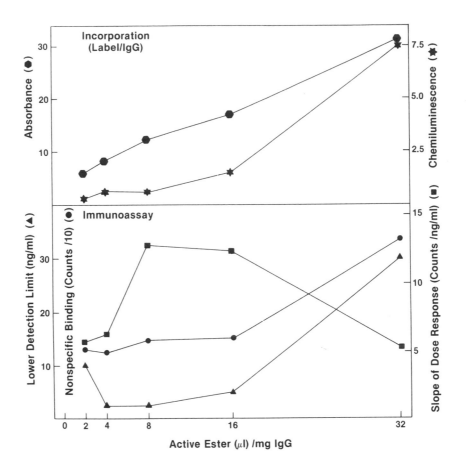

FIG. 7 Correlation of extent of labeling of human IgG with CM-AHEI and performance of conjugates in a sandwich CIA for anti-human IgG. The CIA was performed in plates coated at 2 μg/mL human IgG, otherwise as in Materials and Methods.

The sandwich assay in a microtiter plate was selected because it offers the greatest sensitivity and a convenient format (7,21). The immunoassay for HB_sAg employed conventional conditions and was initiated by adding 100 μL serum specimen manually to the wells coated with anti-HB_sAg. During a 2-h incubation, the antibody bound the HB_sAg. After an intermediate wash step, the sandwich was completed by a 2-h incubation with the chemilumigenic anti-HB_sAg and a final wash step followed. These operations were done simultaneously on 8 or 12 wells at a time using a commercial washer and multipipettor. A luminometer, built in-house, added microperoxidase and peroxide to initiate chemiluminescence and provided automated readout of wells at ten sec intervals. The photon count increased with the amount of chemilumigenic anti-HB_sAg, and was therefore proportional to the HB_sAg levels in the test sample. The model CIA for anti-human IgG followed a similar procedure. However, to insure specificity, excess protein binding sites on human IgG coated wells had to be saturated with BSA.

Both CIAs were optimized. The slopes of dose-response curves in the CIA for HB$_s$Ag increased rapidly as the coating level of partially purified anti-Hb$_s$Ag rose to 20 µg/mL, but remained constant at greater concentrations to 100 µg/mL (Fig. 8). In contrast, with the model CIA slopes were greatest at coating levels of only 0.2-0.5 µg/mL of human IgG and declined quickly with more protein. The optimum amount of chemilumigenic conjugate used to complete the sandwich was determined emperically from the non-specific binding and the dose response. Non-specific binding was reduced to one-third by including BSA at 15% in the PBS diluent for the labeled conjugate. Both optimized CIAs gave a broad dose response from 2-1000 ng/mL (Fig. 9). Vertical bars indicate the standard deviation of the mean photon count (n=6). The detection limit for HB$_s$Ag improved to 1 ng/mL when the incubation with sample was increased to 16 h.

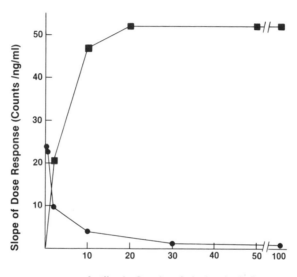

Antibody Coating Solution (µg/ml)

FIG. 8 Effect of antibody concentration for coating plates on the sandwich CIAs for HB$_s$Ag and anti-human IgG. Plates were coated at indicated levels of anti-HB$_s$Ag (■) or human IgG (●) and the human IgG-isoluminol conjugate was used at 0.6 µg/mL where appropriate, otherwise as in Materials and Methods.

The sensitivity and specificity of the CIA for HB$_s$Ag was compared to that of a radioimmunoassay as reference (CLINIRIA[®], Miles Laboratories, Inc.). The detection limits by endpoint dilution of two HB$_s$Ag positive sera (Ad subtype, Center for Blood Research, USA and Paul Ehrlich Institute, West Germany) were 25,000 for both sera in the CIA and 10,000 and 50,000 in the RIA, respectively. Another positive serum (Ay subtype, CBR) gave a detectable response at 4000-fold dilution in both assays. The CIA and RIA correctly identified HB$_s$Ag positive members of the Bureau of Biologics (BOB) panels in the A, B and C category and the negatives (N), which are required for third generation assays (Table 1). In addition, the CIA detected HB$_s$Ag in two to four sera of group (C) and one to two of group D, which are difficult to identify by most RIAs as well. All samples positive for HB$_s$Ag by CIA were confirmable by neutralization testing. When 204

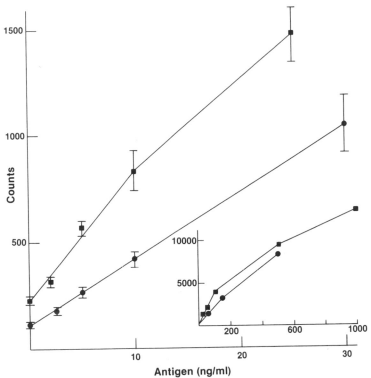

FIG. 9   Sandwich CIAs for HB$_S$Ag in serum (■) and antihuman IgG (●).

TABLE 1.   Comparison of CIA and RIA methods in detecting HB$_S$Ag in Bureau of Biologics HB$_S$Ag Panels 3 and 3A

| Panel | Correct Results/Total Samples | |
	CIA	RIA
A	4/4	4/4
B	10/10	10/10
C	17/17	17/17
(C)	2/7	0/7
D	1/6	0/6
N	6/6	6/6

clinical donor samples were tested in the CIA, 39 were found HB$_S$Ag positive and 37 in a repeat assay (confirmable). These 37 samples and one in addition, were also positive and confirmed in the RIA procedures. The CIA had a false positive rate of about 1% which is typical of various commercial RIAs. The specificity of the CIA was substantiated when similar assays performed in uncoated wells or in wells coated with 25 µg/mL human IgG or BSA produced no dose response with HB_sAg.

The precision of the CIA was established with various dilutions of the PEI standard during a nine-week period. The intra-assay (n=6) and inter-assay (n=4 or 7) variability of photon counts was generally 7-13% CV (Table 2). Despite some scatter these results indicated acceptable reproducibility.

TABLE 2. Reproducibility of the CIA for HB_sAg[a]

HB_sAg (ng/mL)	Inter-Assay (n = 6)[a]		1 Day (n=4)[b]		50 Days (n=7)[b,c]	
	x	% C.V.	x	% C.V.	x	% C.V.
0	179	12	177	10	163	12
1	204	8	199	7	194	11
2	245	10	239	7	211	7
5	361	10	373	10	306	10
10	557	13	515	11	483	11
25	1118	10	1089	13	972	10
50	1817	13	1876	12	1711	11

[a]Six replicates were run in the CIA with the various levels of HB_sAg (PEI standard) as in Materials and Methods.
[b]Values represent the mean of means of six replicates.
[c]Incubation periods of 1.5 h rather than 2 h were used.

The stability of reagents was briefly evaluated. The chemilumigenic anti-HB_sAg conjugate (113 µg/mL) was stored in 15% normal human serum -15% normal rabbit serum - 25 mM Tris-HCl - 250 mM NaCl 0.1% NaN_3, pH 8.6 and 4°C. Its performance in the CIA indicated that the conjugate was stable throughout the four months period tested (Table 3). By comparison, the shelf-life of ^{125}I-labeled anti-HB_sAg is less than two months. Microperoxidase and peroxide were also stable for at least two months (12).

TABLE 3. Stability of the chemilumigenic anti-HB_sAg Conjugate as estimated by performance in the CIA

	Storage (Months)				
	0	1	2	3	4
NC[a]	162	150	161	151	177
NC + 4 SD[b]	190	230	245	235	217
Slope of Dose Response[c]	33	30	28	34	31

[a]The mean photon count for six replicates in the CIA with 1.5 h incubations.
[b]Cut-off value.
[c]Counts/(ng/mL) of HB_sAg.

These results show that the CIA is a valid analytical technique to determine $HB_S Ag$ in serum. It has similar sensitivity and specificity as one RIA, but avoids the stability problems and inconvenience of radio-labels. In contrast to enzyme immunoassays (21), chemiluminescence measurements cover a greater dynamic range and eliminate the need for incubation with substrate, temperature control and a stop reagent.

In conclusion, for practial application, the precision and conven-ience of chemiluminescence measurements need to be improved. Never-theless, chemilumigenic labels are viable alternatives to radiolabels for monitoring immunoassays. Homogeneous CIA procedures are possible, and may have application where only moderate sensitivity is needed. However, a heterogeneous procedure is preferable because it eliminates interference problems from the sample and takes greater advantage of the sensitivity inherent in the chemilumigenic labels. As we have shown, with appropriate instrumentation heterogeneous CIAs can be highly convenient. An important, less obvious advantage of CIAs is that the monitoring reaction takes only a few seconds. Thus, the CIA approach may reduce assay time substantially and merits special consid-eration for mass screening applications requiring high sensitivity.

ACKNOWLEDGEMENTS

I would like to thank C. Hines, D. Osborn, R. Moore, F. Yeager, R. Boguslaski, R. Buckler, P. Vogelhut, and many others at Miles Laboratories who supported these studies.

REFERENCES

1. Burd, J. F., Carrico, R. J., Fetter, M. C., Buckler, R. T., Johnson, R. D., Boguslaski, R. C., and Christner, J. E. (1977): Specific protein-binding reactions monitored by enzymatic hydrol-ysis of ligand-fluorescent dye conjugates. Anal. Biochem., 77:56-67.

2. Carrico, R. J., Yeung, K.-K., Schroeder, H. R., Boguslaski, R. C., Buckler, R. T., and Christner, J. E. (1976): Specific protein-binding reactions monitored with ligand-ATP conjugates and firefly luciferase. Anal. Biochem., 76:95-110.

3. Hersh, S. L., Vann, W. P., and Wilhelm, S. A. (1979): A luminol-assisted competitive-binding immunoassay of human immunoglobulin G. Anal. Biochem., 93:267-271.

4. Kohen, F., Pazzagli, M., Kim, J. B., Lindner, H. R., and Boguslaski, R. C. (1979): An assay procedure for plasma progesterone based on antibody-enhanced chemiluminescence. FEBS Letters, 104:201-205.

5. Ling, C. M., and Overby, L. R. (1972): Prevalance of hepatitis B virus antigen as revealed by direct radioimmune assay with ^{125}I-antibody. J. Immun., 109:834-841.

6. Lowry, OH, Rosebrough, N. J., Farr, A. L., and Randall, R. J. (1951): Protein measurement with the Folin Phenol reagent. J. Biol. Chem., 193:265-275.

7. Purcell, R. H., Wong, D. C., Alter, H. J., and Holland, P. V. (1973): Microtiter solid-phase radioimmunoassay for hepatitis B antigen. Appl. Microbiol., 26:478-484.

8. Rubenstein, K. E., Schneider, R. S., Ullman, E. F. (1972): Homogeneous enzyme immunoassay. A new immunochemical technique. Biochem. Biophys. Res. Commun., 47:846-851.

9. Schroeder, H. R., Carrico, R. J., Boguslaski, R. C., and Christner, J. E. (1976): Specific binding reactions monitored with ligand-cofactor conjugates and bacterial luciferase. Anal. Biochem., 72:283-292.

10. Schroeder, H. R., Vogelhut, P. O., Carrico, R. J., Boguslaski, R. C., and Buckler, R. T. (1976): Competitive protein binding assay for biotin monitored by chemiluminescence. Anal. Chem., 48:1933-1936.

11. Schroeder, H. R., and Yeager, F. M. (1978): Chemiluminescence yields and detection limits of some isoluminol derivatives in various oxydation systems. Anal. Chem., 50: 1114-1120.

12. Schroeder, H. R., Boguslaski, R. C., Carrico, R. J., and Buckler, R. T. (1978): Monitoring specific protein-binding reactions with chemiluminescence. In: Meth. in Enzymol., edited by M. A. DeLuca and W. D. McElroy, pp. 424-445. Academic Press, New York.

13. Schroeder, H. R. and Vogelhut, P. O. (1979): Flow system for sensitive and reproducible chemiluminescence measurements. Anal. Chem., 51:1583-1585.

14. Schroeder, H. R., Yeager, F. M., Boguslaski, R. C., and Vogelhut, P. O. (1979): Immunoassay for serum thyroxine monitored by chemiluminescence. J. Immun. Meth., 25:275-282.

15. Schroeder, H. R., Hines, C. M., Osborn, D. D., Moore, R. P., Hurtle, R. L., Wogoman, F. F., Rogers, R. W., and Vogelhut, P. O. (1981): Immunochemiluminometric assay for hepatitis B surface antigen. Clin. Chem., in press.

16. Schurrs, A. H. W. M. and VanWeeman, B. K. (1977): Enzyme-immunoassay. Clin. Chim. Acta, 81:1-40.

17. Simpson, J. S. A., Campbell, A. K., Ryall, M. E. T., and Woodhead, J. S. (1979): A stable chemiluminescent-labeled antibody for immunological assays. Nature, 279:646-647.

18. Watson, R. A. A., Landon, J., Shaw, E. J., and Smith, D. S. (1976): Polarization fluoroimmunoassay of gentamicin. Clin. Chim. Acta, 73:51-55.

19. Whitehead, T. P., Kricka, L. J., Carter, T. J. N., and Thorpe, G. H. G. (1979): Analytical luminescence: its potential in the clinical laboratory. Clin. Chem., 25: 1531-1546.

20. Wisdom, G. B. (1976): Enzyme-immunoassay. Clin. Chem., 22:1243-1255.

21. Wolters, G., Kuijpers, L. P. C., Kacaki, J. and Schurrs, A. H. W. M. (1977): Enzyme-linked immunosorbent assay for hepatitis B surface antigen. J. Infect. Dis., 136:S311-S317.

Luminescent Assays: Perspectives in Endocrinology and Clinical Chemistry, edited by M. Serio and M. Pazzagli, Raven Press, New York © 1982.

Chemiluminescence Labelled Antibodies and Their Applications in Immunoassays

J. S. Woodhead, I. Weeks, A. K. Campbell, M. E. T. Ryall, *R. Hart, *A. Richardson, and *F. McCapra

*Department of Medical Biochemistry, Welsh National School of Medicine, Cardiff; and *School of Molecular Sciences, Sussex University, Falmer, Sussex, United Kingdom*

Radioimmunoassay has become the method of choice, and in many cases the only method, for the quantitation of a large variety of biologically important molecules. The specificity and high reaction energy of antibodies as binding reagents have led to their widespread *in vitro* use in the precise measurement of compounds present in complex biological fluids at sub-picomolar concentrations. Nevertheless, the methodology of radioimmunoassay has several inherent disadvantages. In the first place, many antigens (e.g. peptide hormones) are difficult to lable with ^{125}I by conventional techniques, and when labelled have relatively short shelf-lives. Secondly, the working range is often limited, thus making optimization difficult. Finally, the need for sensitivity in many polypeptide assays involves the use of reagents at high dilutions, such that reaction times and counting times are inconveniently extended.

In contrast, the immunoradiometric assay (1) and its related procedures (2) utilize labelled antibodies under conditions of reagent excess. Assays using reagent excess attain greater sensitivity with shorter reaction times than conventional radioimmunoassay (3). Moreover, labelled antibodies may be stable for extended periods of time (2), and due to the chemically similar nature of IgG antibodies, universal labelling procedures can be adopted. Nevertheless, even when ^{125}I-labelled antibodies are used, the stability of the label is relatively poor when compared with many of the non-isotopic labels developed in recent years. Indeed, it is the long term stability of enzyme or fluorescent labels that has important advantages in the control of assay performance and makes their use so attactive. In some cases it has

been possible to develop homogeneous assays, requiring no separation
stage, in which the properties of the label are altered when the antigen
binds to antibody.   However, the detection limits of non-isotopic
labels are universally poor when compared with ^{125}I.   For example, with
conventional equipment it is difficult to quantify less than 10^{-13} mol
of fluorescein whereas as little as 10^{-18} mol ^{125}I can be quantified
by γ-counting.

Chemiluminescent molecules possess the advantages of non-isotopic
labels in that they are stable, readily available and can be coupled to
proteins for use in immunoassay systems (4).   In addition, they have a
high sensitivity of detection which suggests their enormous potential
for the development of non-isotopic polypeptide assays.

CHEMILUMINESCENCE

Chemiluminescence is observed when the electronically excited
product of an exoergic reaction reverts to its ground state with photonic
emission.   All the chemiluminescent reactions studied so far are
oxidative, involving a range of organic molecules, the best known of
these being luminol (5-amino-2,3-dihydrophthalazine-1,4-dione).   Luminol
is oxidized by a mixture of hydrogen peroxide, alkali and a catalyst
(e.g. sodium hypochlorite, transition metal ions, peroxidase) (5).   We
have shown previously that a diazonium salt of luminol can be coupled
to antibody protein (4).   Though the quantum yield of the luminol was
greatly reduced following diazotization, the labelled derivative showed
no loss of immunoreactivity and was stable for many months.

Recently, we have studied the use of acridinium esters as potential
labels for immunoassay systems.   These compounds have certain
advantages over luminol.   In particular they can be stimulated to
produce luminescence under relatively mild conditions, requiring
hydrogen peroxide and dilute alkali only (6).   Figure 1 illustrates the
chemiluminescent reaction of an acridinium ester.

Chemiluminescent compounds lose activity slowly under alkaline
conditions due to the presence of endogenous peroxide in aqueous

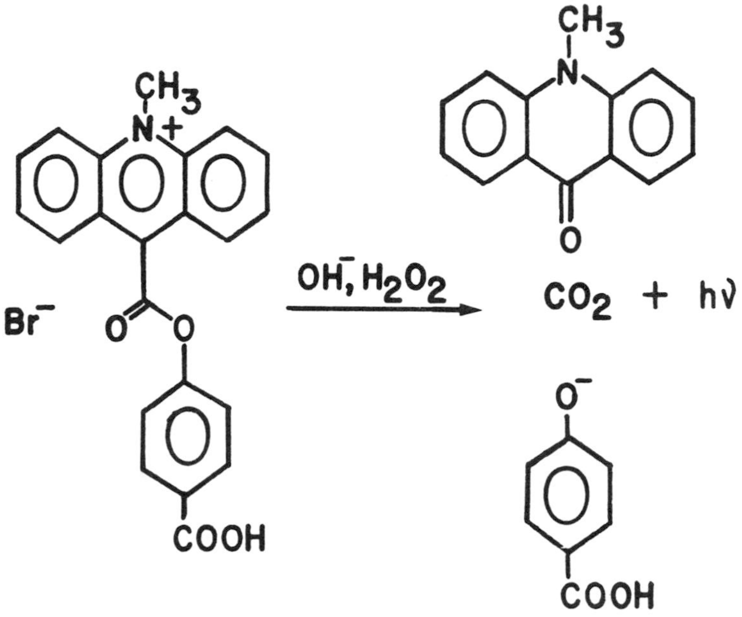

Fig. 1.   Chemiluminescent reaction of an acridinium ester.

solution.   Thus labelled derivatives should be stored at a pH below
7.0 and buffered as required for immunoassay purposes.

LUMINOMETRY

Recent interest in chemiluminescence and bioluminescence as
analytical tools has led to the production of several commercially
available luminometers.   We have built a luminometer in our own
laboratory which takes the following form.   The reaction tube is placed
in front of a photomultiplier (PMT) in a light-tight housing, the PMT
being powered by a stabilized EHT supply.   The PMT amplified emission
from the chemiluminescent reaction can be fed to a scalar for
integration.   Alternatively the rate at which photons arrive at the
photocathode can be displayed on an oscilloscope or chart recorder
following storage in a transient recorder.

Following initiation of the chemiluminescent reaction, light

emission rises rapidly, reaches a peak and then decays with simple first
order kinetics, the time constant for the decay phase being a function
of the concentration of peroxide (5). This reagent dependence of the
reaction rate enables conditions to be chosen such that the photons
generated by the reaction can be quantified very rapidly. The ability
to quantify label rapidly offers a major advantage over radioisotope
measurement, where the counting system may limit the rate at which
assays can be carried out.

PREPARATION OF LABELLED ANTIBODIES

While reagent excess assays are relatively simple to carry out, the
preparation of the reagents may be more demanding than for conventional
radioimmunoassay. For the immunoradiometric assay, antibodies are
first purified from antiserum by affinity chromatography and labelled
with ^{125}I while still bound to the solid phase (2). Because of the
ready availability of chemiluminescent molecules, it is possible to
label IgG preparations, which contain relatively small proportions of
specific antibody, and then carry out purification by affinity chromatography. This latter practice has been adopted for the studies reported
here.

As described above, initial studies with luminol labelled antibodies (4) established that stable, immunoreactive derivatives could be
produced though the quantum yield of the chemiluminescent reaction was
disappointing. Subsequent experiments were carried out using a
succinyl derivative of luminol which was reacted with sheep (anti-rabbit
IgG) antibodies by either mixed anhydride or carbodiimide coupling
procedures (7). Though the incorporation in both cases was lower, the
specific activity of the labelled antibody was similar to that obtained
by diazotization. It proved difficult, however, to obtain incorporations of label better than 1 mol luminol/mol IgG.

Preliminary experiments with acridinium esters suggest that the
chemiluminescent reaction is not adversely affected by derivatization
for coupling. Studies in which sheep antibodies to human α-fetoprotein
(AFP) were labelled with p-carboxyphenyl-N,10-methylacridinium-9-

carboxylate bromide using carbodiimide yielded labelled antibodies of high luminescent activity despite relatively low incorporations of the chemiluminescent molecule (7).

We have recently investigated more convenient coupling methods using derivatives which react spontaneously with protein rather than reacting protein and chemiluminescent compound simultaneously with a coupling reagent.   Derivatives of acridinium esters which form stable amide bonds with primary and secondary amines incorporate readily into protein under mild conditions as shown in Table 1.

Table 1.   Incorporation of acridinium ester into rabbit IgG.

Time (min)	Incorporation (counts/mol IgG)
10	3.5×10^{15}
100	1.38×10^{16}
250	1.43×10^{16}
500	1.50×10^{6}

After 10 minutes at pH 7.0 there was significant uptake of label into rabbit IgG, using a ratio of acridinium derivative to protein of 2:1.   The reaction was stopped by quenching with lysine followed by extensive dialysis.   An IgG preparation of sheep-(anti AFP) antibodies was similarly labelled and purified labelled antibody isolated by extensive dialysis and affinity chromatography using solid phase AFP.

ASSAYS WITH CHEMILUMINESCENT LABELS

Acridinium ester labelled rabbit IgG was used in a system analogous to conventional radioimmunoassay.   Label and standards were reacted for 18 h with a solid phase antibody consisting of a sheep-(anti rabbit IgG) preparation linked covalently to reprecipitated cellulose.   Separation was by centrifugation and the bound label quantified by chemiluminescent reaction.

A standard curve for this assay is shown in Figure 2.   Though

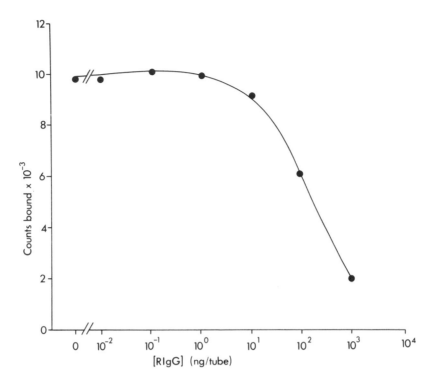

Fig. 2.   Solid phase chemiluminescent immunoassay of rabbit IgG.

Two - site Immunoassay

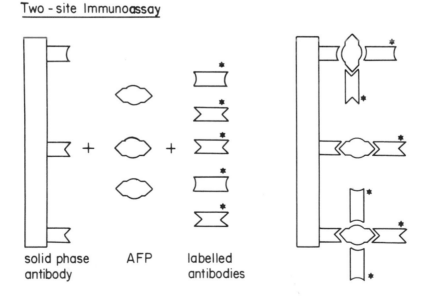

solid phase   AFP   labelled
antibody   antibodies

Fig. 3.   Two site luminometric assay protocol.

assay conditions were not rigorously optimised, sensitivity was similar to that obtained using ^{125}I-labelled rabbit IgG.

A two site assay of human AFP was set up using the protocol outlined in Fig. 3. Standards were reacted simultaneously with cellulose-linked sheep-(anti AFP) antibody and labelled antibody for 1 h at room temperature. After centrifugation the bound chemiluminescence was measured. The standard curve (Fig. 4) shows uptake of label as a function of AFP concentration, which exhibits the so-called high dose hook effect frequently seen in this type of assay (8).

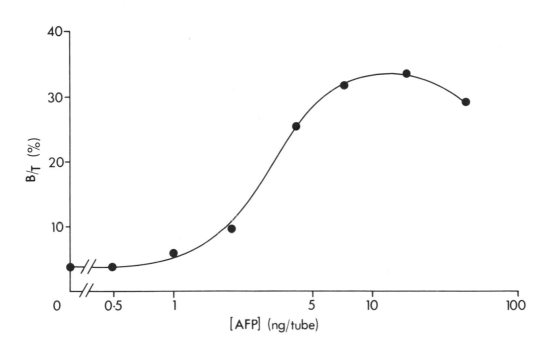

Fig. 4. Standard curve for two-site luminometric assay of AFP.

DISCUSSION

Chemiluminescent molecules fulfil the criteria for use as labels in immunoassay. They are readily available and can be quantified using relatively simple equipment. As these experiments show, they can be coupled to protein to produce stable derivatives, which retain both

chemiluminescent and immunological activity.   Their unique advantage
over other non-isotopic labels is their high sensitivity of detection,
acridinium esters being readily quantified in amounts as little as
10^{-17} mol or less.

Labelled antibody assays offer advantages over conventional radioimmunoassay techniques in terms of specificity (9) and also speed and
sensitivity (3).   The use of excess binding reagent produces rapid
reactions, where sensitivity is less dependent on affinity or the
specific activity of the label.   We have shown, for example, when
label incorporation is low, it is still possible to develop two-site
assays for AFP capable of measuring the antigen in the clinically useful
range.

While the preparation of labelled antibody reagents has proved
demanding in the past due to the requirement for affinity purification
with solid phase antigen, it is likely that these difficulties will now
be overcome by the increasing availability of monoclonal antibodies to
biologically important molecules.

The performance of conventional immunoassays is ultimately limited
by the affinity of the antibody for the antigen.   This restriction
does not apply to labelled antibody assays using reagent excess.   Thus
improvements in luminometry and hence the detection limits for chemiluminescent molecules will lead to the development of luminometric
assays of polypeptides with considerably improved sensitivity.

Acknowledgements

This work has been supported by grants from the Department of
Health and Social Security, the Science Research Council and the
Medical Research Council.

References

1.   Miles, L.E.M. and Hales, C.N. (1968) Nature 219, 136 - 189

2.   Woodhead, J.S., Addison, G.M. and Hales, C.N. (1974) Brit. Med.

Bull. <u>30</u>, 44 – 49

3.   Kemp, H.A., Simpson, J.S.A. and Woodhead, J.S. (1981) Clin. Chem. in press

4.   Simpson, J.S.A., Campbell, A.K., Ryall, M.E.T. and Woodhead, J.S. (1979) Nature <u>279</u>, 646 – 647

5.   White, E.H. and Brendett, R.B. (1973) In Chemiluminescence and Bioluminescence (Ed. Cormier, M.J., Hercules, E.M. and Lee, J.) Plenum, New York, pp 231 – 244

6.   McCapra, F., Tutt, D.E. and Topping R.M. British Patent No. 1,461,877

7.   Simpson, J.S.A., Campbell, A.K., Woodhead, J.S., Richardson, A., Hart, R. and McCapra, F. (1981) In Bioluminescence and Chemiluminescence (Ed. DeLuca, M. and McElroy, W.D.) Academic Press, pp 673 – 679

8.   Miles, L.E.M., Lipschitz, D.A., Bieber, C.P. and Cook, J.D. (1974) Anal. Biochem. <u>61</u>, 209 – 224

9.   Rainbow, S.J., Woodhead, J.S., Yue, D.K., Luzio, S.D. and Hales, C.N. (1979) Diabetologia <u>17</u>, 229 – 234.

Luminescent Assays: Perspectives in Endocrinology and Clinical Chemistry, edited by M. Serio and M. Pazzagli, Raven Press, New York © 1982.

Enzyme Immunoassays Using Horseradish Peroxidase as a Label Assayed by Chemiluminescence with Luminol Derivatives as Substrates

*K.-D. Gundermann, K. Wulff, R. Linke, and F. Stähler

Boehringer Mannheim GmbH, Research Center Tutzing, 8132 Tutzing, Federal Republic of Germany;
Organisch-Chemisches Institut, Technische Universität Clausthal, 3392 Clausthal-Zellerfeld,
Federal Republic of Germany

The development of the method of radioimmunoassays by Berson and Yalow (2) had been a great breakthrough in trace analysis. Since a few years, however, more and more problems arise with the handling of radioactive waste. Hence many attempts were made to find non-radioactive labels for immunoassays providing a similar sensitivity as the radioactive ones. One of the most important achievments has been the development of immunoassays using horseradish peroxidase as a label (1).

Several attempts have been made to develop immunoassays by using luminescent labels, e.g. luminol or luminol derivatives (6,7,9,11,12), substrates of bioluminescence reactions like ATP (3) or NAD (10), or firefly luciferase (13).

In 1976 Puget and Michelson (8) demonstrated that horseradish peroxidase is able to catalyze the oxidation of 3-aminophthalic hydrazide (luminol) by hydrogen peroxide showing a chemiluminescence. However, this method does not provide an assay for horseradish peroxidase as sensitive as the assay using the chromogenic substrate 2.2'-azino-di-3-ethyl-benthiazoline-sulfonate (6).

Gundermann and coworkers (4,5) synthesized several derivatives of luminol, which in alkaline solution with heme as catalyst show a significantly higher quantum yield compared with luminol.

In this communication we are presenting data on a system for comparing the effectiveness of chemiluminescent peroxidase substrates as well as on a chemiluminescence immunoassay composed of a commercially available enzymeimmunoassay using a luminol derivative as substrate.

MATERIALS AND METHODS

Luminol and luminol derivatives have been synthesized according to published procedures (4,5). The emzymeimmunoassay testkit, Enzymun Test(R) Digoxin (cat.no 199656) was from Boehringer Mannheim. All other chemicals were of reagent grade, either from Boehringer Mannheim or from Merck, Darmstadt.

Chemiluminescence assays were performed using an ATP- photometer 3000 of SAI, San Diego, Cal. The signal was followed with a recorder and the light intensity between the 2nd and 5th minute after starting the reaction was integrated graphically giving relative light units.

The luminol derivatives were tested in the following way: A scintillation vial contained in 2.0 ml: o,2 mmol potassium phosphate buffer pH 7.0, 200 nmol EDTA, 1 μg horseradish peroxidase, variable amounts of the compound tested, and 24 nmol hydrogen peroxide. The reaction was started by the addition of the peroxide. The light emission was measured as indicated above.

The chemiluminescence digoxin assay was done in the following way:

The immunological part of the reaction was performed according to the recommendations of the manufacturer. Then 1 ml of a solution containing 100 nmol 7-dimethylamino naphthalene-1.2-dicarbonic acid hydrazide, 0.1 mmol potassium phosphate, pH 8.2, 100 nmol EDTA, and 120 nmol hydrogen peroxide was placed into the vial and the light emission followed on the recorder. The light intensity was integrated as mentioned above.

RESULTS AND DISCUSSION

As can be seen in Fig. 1 the light intensities measured in a pure system composed of horseradish peroxidase, hydrogen peroxide, salts and the luminescent substrate can be plotted analogue to a Michaelis-Menten plot giving a rate parameter I_{max} and an affinity parameter K_m.

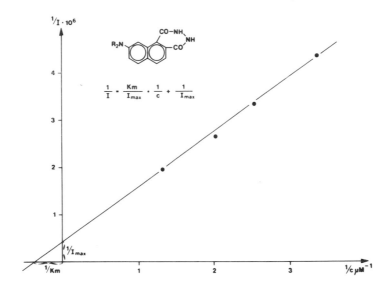

Fig. 1. Reciprocal plot of relative light intensity units against substrate concentration.

Table 1 shows these parameters for luminol and its derivatives compared with the relative quantum yields in the heme-catalyzed reaction. The highest quantum yield in heme catalysis gives the 7-dipropyl-amino-naphthalene-1.2-dicarbonic acid hydrazide, whereas it yields only a poor chemiluminescence in the peroxidase catalyzed reaction, where the 7-dimethyl derivative is the most active one. These differences can be explained considering steric effects at the active site of the peroxidase molecule. Although only those compounds showing an elevated quantum yield in heme catalysis compared with luminol can be considered as potential peroxidase substrates of sufficient sensitivity, this quality cannot be predicted from the quantum yield, exclusively, due to the unknown steric effects.

From the compounds listed in Table 1 the 7-dimethyl-derivative was found to be most active one in the peroxidase assay.

Table 1:

Reaction parameters of luminol and some of its derivatives.

derivative	horse radish peroxidase as catalyst		heme catalysis
	I_{max}	K_m	relative quantum yield
luminol	$6 \cdot 10^5$	$1.3 \cdot 10^{-6}$	1.0
4-diethylamino-phthalic hydrazide	$2.4 \cdot 10^4$	$3.4 \cdot 10^{-6}$	
7-dimethylamino-naphthalene-1.2-dicarbonic acid hydrazide	$3 \cdot 10^6$	$4 \cdot 10^{-6}$	2.3
7-dipropylamino-naphthalene-1.2-dicarbonic acid hydrazide	nearly inactive		3.0

Therefore, we tried this compound as substrate in a commercially available digoxin immunoassay (Fig. 2). To perform this assay with the chromogenic substrate an incubation time for the enzyme reaction of 60 minutes is required. Using the chemiluminescent substrate an

incubation time of only 5 minutes is necessary to get an acceptable
calibration curve (Fig. 2).

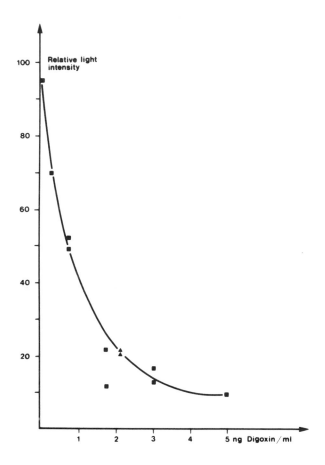

Fig. 2. Calibration curve for Enzymun Test[R] digoxin using 7-di-
         methylamino-naphthalene-1.2-dicarbonic acid hydrazide as
         substrate for horseradish peroxidase assay.

         The triangels repesent digoxin standards.

Similar results have been obtained with enzymeimmuno assays for insulin
and for thyroxine, respectively. Hence the time necessary to get a
result from these assays is shortened by nearly one hour using the
luminol derivative as substrate.
    From these data it may be concluded that an enzyme immunoassay
using horseradish peroxidase as label and 7-dimethylamino-naphthalene-
1.2-dicarbonic acid hydrazide as substrate can be optimized towards
an increased sensitivity of at least 10 times beyond the state of art.

REFERENCES

1. Avrameas, S. (1969): Coupling of enzymes to proteins with glutardialdehyde. Use of the conjugates for the detection of antigens and antibodies. Immunochemistry, 6: 43 - 52

2. Berson, S.A., and Yalow, R.S. (1959): Quantitative aspects of reaction between insulin and insulin-binding antiboby. J. Clin. Invest., 38: 1966 - 2016.

3. Carrico, R.J., Yeung, K.-K., Schroeder, H.R., Boguslaski, R.C., Buckler, R.T., and Christner, J.E. (1976): Specific protein-binding reactions monitored with ligand-ATP conjugates and firefly luciferase. Anal. Biochem., 76: 95 - 110.

4. Gundermann, K.-D., Horstmann, W., Bergmann, G. (1965): Synthese und Chemilumineszenzverhalten von 7-Dialkylamino-naphthalin-dicarbon-säure-(1.2)-hydraziden. Liebigs Ann. Chem., 684: 127 - 141.

5. Gundermann, K.-D., Lathia, D., Nolte, W., and Röker, K.-D. (1974): Einfluß der Substitutionsposition auf die Chemilumineszenz von Benzo[f]phthalazin-1,4 (2H, 3H)-dionen. Liebigs Ann. Chem., 1974: 798 - 808.

6. Hersh, L.S., Vann, W.P., and Wilhelm, S.A. (1979): A luminol-assisted competitive binding immunoassay of human immunoglobulin G. Anal. Biochem., 93: 267 - 271.

7. Kohen, F., Pazzagli, M., Kim, J.B., Lindner, H.R., and Boguslaski, R.C. (1979): An assay procedure for plasma progesterone based on antibody-enhanced chemiluminescence. FEBS-Lett., 104: 201 - 205.

8. Puget, K. and Michelson, A.M. (1976): Microestimation of glucose and glucose oxidase. Biochimie, 58: 757 - 758.

9. Pratt, J.J., Woldring, M.G., and Villerius, L. (1978): Chemiluminescence-linked immunoassay. J. Immunol. Meth., 21:179-184.

10. Schroeder, H.R., Carrico, R.J., Boguslaski, R.C., and Christner, J.E. (1976): Specific binding reactions monitored with ligand-cofactor conjugates and bacterial luciferase. Anal. Biochem., 72: 283 - 292.

11. Schroeder, H.R., Yeager, F.M., Boguslaski, R.C., and Vogelhut, P.O. (1979): Immunoassay for serum thyroxine monitored by chemi-luminescence. J. Immunol. Meth., 25: 275 - 282.

12. Simpson, J.S.A., Campbell, A.K., Ryall, M.E.T., and Woodhead, J.S. (1979): A stable chemiluminescent-labelled antibody for immunological assays. Nature, 279: 646 - 647.

13. Wannlund, J., Azari, J., Levine, L., and DeLuca, M. (1980): A bio-Luminescent immunoassay for methotrexate at the subpicomole level. Biochem. Biophys. Res. Commun. 96: 440 - 446.

Luminescent Assays: Perspectives in Endocrinology and Clinical Chemistry, edited by M. Serio and M. Pazzagli, Raven Press, New York © 1982.

A Chemiluminescent System Used to Increase the Sensitivity in Enzyme Immunoassy

R. Botti, P. Leoncini, P. Tarli, and P. Neri

ISVT Sclavo, Research Centre, 53100 Siena, Italy

Sensitivity is an essential characteristic of every analytical method, determining its field of application. Very often the final determination of enzymatic activity in enzyme immunoassay is performed by colorimetry.

Luminometry can represent a useful alternative, increasing the sensitivity of enzyme immunoassay in comparison with the colorimetric procedure.

The purpose of this paper was to verify whether, by using as tracer an enzyme which could be determined both colorimetrically and luminometrically and by setting up an enzyme immunoassay method with final detection by chemiluminescence, it was possible to obtain an increase in analytical sensitivity.

Of the various enzymes offering the possibility of determination by either colorimetric or luminescent techniques, Glucose oxidase (GOD) was selected. In fact, this enzyme provides reproducible tracers which are stable over a long period of time, and which can be prepared with reactions which have already been described and standardized. Moreover, the conjugates contain a high percentage of added enzymatic activity, maintaining most of the original antibody activity with low background (4,5). In addition, glucose oxidase is an enzyme which develops hydrogen peroxide during a pre-incubation period that is appropriately selected in order to increase the sensitivity of the system.

RESULTS

GOD titrations

Luminescent method

GOD (70 U/mg) was titrated by incubating 20 µl of enzyme solution (ranging from 0.5 to 400 ng/ml) at room temperature for 50 minutes with

200 μl of a solution of glucose substrate (5 mg/ml in 10 mM phosphate buffer pH 7.0).

The hydrogen peroxide developed was determined in a 100 μl aliquot by adding 100 μl of 10 mM Ferricyanide solution and 100 μl of 20 mM Luminol solution in 20 mM Glycine-HCl buffer pH 10.5, using polystyrene lumino-meter cuvettes.

These final steps and the readings were performed using the automatic injection and integration system of a 3-pump Lumac Biocounter Mod. 2010 luminometer. Readings begin 2 seconds after the reaction starts; light emission is then measured for 10 seconds and recorded as arbitrary light units (ALU).

<u>Colorimetric method</u>

GOD titration was performed in polystyrene plates by incubating 20 μl of enzyme solution (at the same concentrations as previously reported) with 200 μl of a solution of glucose (5 mg/ml), peroxidase (50 U/mg; 20 μg/ml) and 2.2'-Azino-di[3-ethyl-benzothiazolin-sulfonate] diammonium salt (ABTS) chromogen (0.5 mg/ml in 100 mM phosphate buffer pH 7.0. After 50 minutes at room temperature, readings of optical density (OD) were performed at 405 nm using a Flow Titertek Multiskan apparatus.

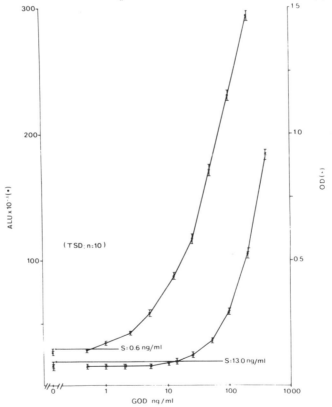

Fig. 1. GOD titration by the chemiluminescent (•) and colorimetric (x) method. Each point represents the mean ± SD of 10 replicates.

Figure 1 reports the results of GOD titrations using the luminescent and colorimetric technique. The luminescent method appears to be more sensitive (about 20 times) than the colorimetric one. In fact, the sensitivity, defined as the dose that is expected to give a response differing by at least two standard deviations from the response for zero dose (1), is 0.6 ng/ml adopting the chemiluminescent method and 13.0 ng/ml when the colorimetric technique is used.

On the basis of these results, we have developed an enzyme immunoassay using GOD as tracer enzyme to determine the sensitivity when monitored by chemiluminescence. A solid phase sandwich technique was adopted in view of its greater sensitivity with respect to the competitive protein binding assay (3,9). Moreover, the washing steps of this technique allow the elimination of substances which could potentially interfere in the chemiluminescent reaction (8). The determination of serum levels of human chorionic somatomammotropin (hCS or hPL) was selected as a model.

Conjugate preparation

The immunoglobulin G fraction (IgG) was isolated from a specific goat anti-hCS serum by ammonium sulphate precipitation, followed by DEAE-cellulose chromatography (10). Coupling with GOD was performed in a molar ratio, using the periodate reaction according to the method of Nakane and Kawaoi (6).

The conjugate was purified by Ultrogel AcA 34 column chromatography and maintained in 1% bovine serum albumin (BSA), 0.01% NaN_3 at 4°C. It is stable under these conditions for at least 6 months.

Each conjugate preparation was characterized by determining the enzymatic and immunological activities remaining after the labelling reaction and column purification.

Preparation of the plates

The immunoassay was performed in 96-well polystyrene plates which had proved useful and convenient in similar procedures (2,11,12). The wells were previously coated by filling with 200 µl of anti-hCS IgG solution (45 µg/ml) in 0.1M sodium carbonate pH 9.8 at 37°C for 3 hours and overnight at 4°C. The wells were washed three times prior to use, in phosphate buffer saline (PBS) containing 0.5% Brij 35 using a Flow Titertek Multiwash apparatus.

Enzyme immunoassay

Different dilutions of an hCS-free serum supplemented with known amounts of hormone were prepared in PBS containing 0.5% Brij 35 and 1% BSA. 200 µl of each solution were added to the wells and incubated at 37°C for 2 hours. After washing (3 times with PBS containing 0.5% Brij and 1% BSA), 200 µl of appropriately diluted conjugate solution were added to each well and incubated for 2 hours at room temperature. The wells were subjected to a final washing step.

The enzymatic detection was performed by a chemiluminescent or colorimetric procedure under the conditions previously described for GOD titration.

Sensitivity and linearity range

A typical reference curve obtained with the chemiluminescent method using 10 replicates for each point is reported in Figure 2 (left side). The sensitivity (1) is 0.0020 ng per tube while the linear part of the curve ranges between about 0.05 and 2 ng per tube.

Using the colorimetric detection technique, the sensitivity is 0.035 ng per tube and the linearity range is between 0.15 and 2 ng per tube (Figure 2, right side).

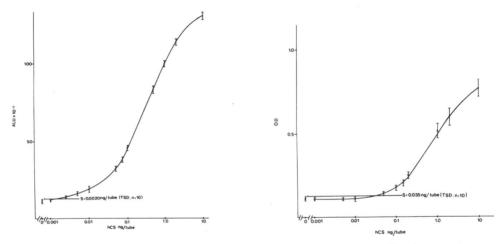

Fig. 2. Reference curves for hCS obtained with the chemiluminescent (left side) and colorimetric (right side) methods. Each point represents the mean $\pm$ SD of 10 replicates.

Precision studies

Precision studies were performed for both techniques using 5 human sera at various stages of pregnancy. The within-assay precision was evaluated by 10 replicate analyses of hCS concentrations in 3 of the sera. The between-assay precision was estimated by performing replicate measurements on the other 2 sera in 6 consecutive assays on different days.

The results show that the coefficients of variation for the chemiminescent technique are lower than for the colorimetric method, particularly at low levels of analyte (Table I).

Correlation with radioimmunoassay

Twentytwo pregnant human sera were assayed for their hCS levels by radioimmunoassay and by chemiluminescent enzyme immunoassay, using the same antiserum. The results obtained in the two methods are in good agreement: $r = 0.986$; $y = 0.25 + 0.94x$ ($\mu g/ml$) where y represents the values determined by the chemiluminescent enzyme immunoassay (Fig. 3).

TABLE 1. Chemiluminescent and colorimetric enzyme immunoassay for hCS: Precision studies

	hCS conc. (µg/ml)		CV %
	mean	SD	
Chemiluminescent determination			
Within-assay: Serum no. 1	0.46	0.03	6.5
" 2	1.90	0.10	5.3
" 3	7.30	0.40	5.5
Between-assay: Serum no. 4	1.12	0.10	8.9
" 5	5.16	0.49	9.5
Colorimetric determination			
Within-assay: Serum no. 1	0.52	0.06	11.5
" 2	2.20	0.21	9.5
" 3	6.95	0.59	8.5
Between-assay: Serum no. 4	0.92	0.14	15.2
" 5	5.60	0.60	10.7

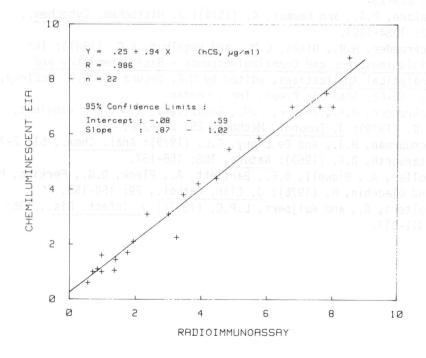

Fig. 3. Correlation of serum hCS levels as determined by radioimmuno-assay and chemiluminescent enzyme immunoassay.

CONCLUSION

The alternative chemiluminescent method proposed appears to increase the sensitivity (and precision) in comparison with the enzyme immuno-assay for hCS determination using a final colorimetric revelation technique.

Obviously this method can be applied to the determination of different analytes, also using other immunoassay techniques. This is of particular importance in view of the possibility of partial or total automation of luminescent measurements (7).

REFERENCES

1. Abraham, G.E. (1974): Acta Endocrinologica, Suppl. 183, 75: 1-42.
2. Bartlett, A., Dormandy, K.M., Hawkey, C.M., Stableforth, P., and Voller, A. (1976): Brit. Med. J., 1: 994-996.
3. Ekins, R. (1981): In: Immunoassays for the 80's, edited by A. Voller, A. Bartlett, and D. Bidwell, pp. 5-16. MTP Press Ltd., Lancaster.
4. Johnson, R.B. Jr., Libby, R.M., and Nakamura, R.M. (1980): J. Immuno. y, 1: 27-37.
5. Maiolini, R., and Masseyeff, R. (1975): J. Immunol. Methods, 8: 223-234.
6. Nakane, P.A., and Kawaoi, A. (1974): J. Histochem. Cytochem., 22: 1084-1091.
7. Schroeder, H.R., Hines, C.M., and Vogelhut, P.O. (1981): In: Bioluminescence and Chemiluminescence - Basic Chemistry and Analytical Applications, edited by M.A. DeLuca and W.D. McElroy, pp. 55-62. Academic Press, Inc., London.
8. Schroeder, H.R., Yeager, F.M., Boguslaski, R.G., and Vogelhut, P.O. (1979): J. Immunol. Methods, 25: 275-282.
9. Schuurman, H.J., and De Ligny, C.L. (1979): Anal. Chem., 51: 2-7.
10. Stanworth, D.R. (1960): Nature, 188: 156-157.
11. Voller, A., Bidwell, D.E., Bartlett, A., Fleck, D.G., Perkins, M., and Oladehin, B. (1976): J. Clin. Pathol., 29: 150-153.
12. Wolters, G., and Kuijpers, L.P.C. (1977): J. Infect. Dis., 136: S311-317.

*Luminescent Assays: Perspectives in
Endocrinology and Clinical Chemistry*, edited by
M. Serio and M. Pazzagli, Raven Press,
New York © 1982.

Steroid Immunoassays Using Chemiluminescent Labels

F. Kohen, J. B. Kim, H. R. Lindner, and *Z. Eshhar

*Department of Hormone Research and *Chemical Immunology, The Weizmann Institute of Science, Rehovot 76100, Israel*

The diagnosis of endocrine disorders requires the determination of hormones or of specific hormone metabolites in body fluids. In blood plasma, the hormone to be measured may be present in minute concentrations, often in the presence of much higher concentration of chemically related but hormonally inert substances. Hence highly sensitive and specific methods are required. To be clinically useful, these should be cheap, rapid and reliable. Radioimmunoassay (RIA) provides the most practical approach to achieve this and has penetrated every major hospital laboratory. Although RIA is sensitive, reasonably specific and convenient, it possesses certain disadvantages inherent in the use of radioactive labels, such as the problem of radioactive waste disposal, and the relatively short shelf-life of the iodinated tracers. Furthermore, RIA procedures depend on the availability of a suitable radiolabeled ligand and of expensive equipment. Recent studies from our laboratory (8-11) and elsewhere (14,18-21) have shown that chemiluminescence immunoassay can be a feasible alternative to RIA of steroids. The steroid-chemiluminescent marker conjugates have been shown to be stable, and can be measured at pM levels (8-12). We report here the use of these labels in the development of various formats of chemiluminescent based steroid immunoassays. These include "homogeneous" methods not requiring a phase separation step (8-11), and heterogeneous methods utilizing dextran-coated charcoal (15-17) or solid-phase separation system (2-4,12). These methods are assessed for specificity, sensitivity accuracy and precision and for monitoring ovarian function in the clinical laboratory. In addition, we describe here the use of monoclonal antibody preparations (4,5) in the standardization of the assays.

MATERIALS AND METHODS

Phthalhydrazide derivatives such as 6[N-(4-aminobutyl)-N-ethyl]-amino-2,3-dihydrophthalazine-1,4-dione (aminobutyl ethyl isoluminol, ABEI), aminopentyl ethyl isoluminol (APEI), aminohexyl ethyl isoluminol (AHEI) were synthesized according to published procedures (20) and were conjugated through a peptide bond to carboxy derivatives of steroids [e.g., progesterone-11α-hemisuccinate (7), cortisol-21-hemisuccinate, estriol-6(0)-carboxymethyl oxime (7)] and steroid glucuronides [estriol-16α-glucuronide (9), estrone-3-glucuronide and pregnanediol-3α-glucuronide (4)] to yield the corresponding steroid-chemiluminescent marker conjugates. A two-step reaction method via an activated ester was used for the condensation of carboxyl derivatives of steroids with amino derivatives of isoluminol (9,10).

Anti-steroidal IgG fractions were prepared by chromatography on Sepharose-Protein-A (9,10). The production of monoclonal antibodies to steroid hormones (4,5), the reagents for immunoassay, and the development of both homogeneous and heterogeneous (e.g., solid-phase) chemiluminescence based immunoassay procedures were as previously described (12), unless specified otherwise.

Measurements of light emission were made with Luminometer Model 2080 (Lumac Systems, Basel), using the automatic injection and integration modes of the instrument, and were recorded as arbitrary light units.

DEVELOPMENT OF HOMOGENEOUS IMMUNOASSAYS BASED ON CHEMILUMINESCENCE

Effect of homologous antibody on the light yield during oxidation of
steroid-chemiluminescent marker conjugates

The steroid-chemiluminescent marker conjugates produced light upon oxidation by a hydrogen peroxide-microperoxidase system at pH 8.6. Light emission measured 2 sec after addition of oxidant increased linearly with steroid-chemiluminescent marker conjugate concentration and the lower limit of detection was 4 pg/tube (9-11). When the steroid-chemiluminescent marker conjugates were bound to the homologous anti-steroid antibodies, three types of antibody-induced effects on the light yield of the steroid-chemiluminescent marker conjugates during oxidation were observed:-

i) in the progesterone (8,11) and estriol-16α-glucuronide systems (9), the homologous antibody caused an increase in both the peak light of light emission and the total light yield of the steroid-chemiluminescent marker conjugate during oxidation;

ii) in the cortisol system (10), the homologous antibody did not augment the peak height of the light response of cortisol-APEI conjugate during oxidation, but on the contrary, reduced and total light yield was only slightly increased; however, the antibody caused a delay in light emission, resulting in a shift of the response curve to the right;

iii) in the estriol system (9), monoclonal antibody generated with 17β-estradiol-6(0)-carboxymethyl oxime bovine serum albumin with a high cross reaction for estriol (50%) enhanced total light yield of estriol-APEI conjugate, with no significant effect on peak height.

In all three systems addition of unaltered homologous steroid to the reaction inhibited the light production. In the first system, a reduction in both the peak height of light emission and total light yield was observed (Fig. 1). In the second system, addition of free cortisol prevented the shift of the light emission to the right (10). In the third system, addition of free estriol did not reduce the peak height of light emission, but a reduction of total light yield was seen (9). The antibody effect on the light emission of the steroid-chemiluminescent marker conjugate during oxidation thus formed the basis of

of each assay system.

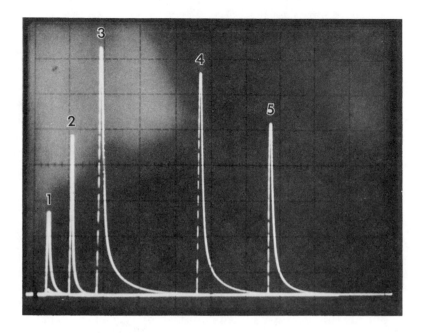

FIG. 1. Oscilloscope tracings of the light signal obtained upon
oxidation of progesterone-ABEI conjugate in the presence of
specific antibody with or without addition of progesterone.
Legend: (1) signal obtained when the enzyme solution only was
mixed with the oxidant at pH 8.6; (2) signal due to the oxidation
of 40 pg of progesterone-ABEI conjugate; (3) signal obtained when
the conjugate (40 pg) was oxidized in the presence of anti-progesterone IgG (0.034 pmol/tube); (4) and (5) signals obtained
when the conjugate (40 pg) was oxidized in the presence of anti-
progesterone - IgG (0.034 pmol) and progesterone (62 pg and 625
pg respectively). Scale used on the oscilloscope : speed 2 sec/
1.22 cm; sensitivity : 4 x 100mV/1.22 cm.

Development of assay procedures for steroids and steroid glucuro-
nides based on monitoring chemiluminescence

Dose response curves for estriol-16α-glucuronide (9), for
progesterone (8,11), for cortisol (10) and for estriol (11) were
assembled by using the steroid-chemiluminescent marker conjugate,
the homologous antibody to the steroid and the homologous unaltered steroid as the competitor. The range of the dose-response
curve was similar to that obtained by RIA procedures (10 - 100 pg
or 20 - 1,000 pg/tube), and a phase-separation was not necessary.
The progesterone assay was refined by studying the influence of
length of spacer between the steroid and isoluminol on the light
yield (11).

The chemiluminescence immunoassays for these steroids were
validated in terms of specificity, sensitivity, linear range,

precision and reproducibility. Procedures were established for preparing biological samples [plasma (9-11) and urine extracts (9)] for assays, and assay results were correlated with those substances by RIA procedures.

Remarks

In each system described above, the antibody effect on the light yield of the homologous steroid-chemiluminescent marker conjugate during oxidation forms the basis of the assay. Thus, we do not know whether the observed antibody effect is a peculiar property of the particular steroid conjugate used as a labeled ligand or is due to the type of antibody employed in the assay. It would appear that the detailed assay procedure will have to be adopted in each case to the type of antibody used, or else the antibody to be used will have to be rigidly standardized, e.g., by using the hybridoma technique (13).

Moreover, the homogeneous assay procedure was affected by interference from luminescent compounds present in extracts of plasma or diluted urine samples (9). To overcome this problem, several procedures have been attempted. These include ion-exchange chromatography of diluted urine (9), solvent extraction followed by a phase separation using dextran-coated charcoal (14,17) and solid-phase techniques (2,3). The results of heterogeneous immunoassays based on chemiluminescence are reported in the sections following.

DEVELOPMENT OF HETEROGENEOUS IMMUNOASSAYS BASED ON MONITORING
CHEMILUMINESCENCE

Separation of bound and free forms of the ligand with dextran-coated charcoal

Dextran-coated charcoal is commonly used in RIA of steroid hormones. Taking this fact into consideration, chemiluminescence based immunoassays were developed for cortisol (15) and progesterone (16,17), using dextran-coated charcoal for separation of bound and free forms of the ligand. The light yield of the bound conjugate was then determined by oxidation with a H_2O_2-microperoxidase system at pH 13. Assay curves for these steroids were obtained with a range of 15-1,000 pg steroid/assay tube. Fig. 2 shows a typical dose-response curve for cortisol. Using this system, assay procedures for determination of plasma progesterone (17) and of plasma and urinary free cortisol (15) were established after a preliminary extraction step of the biological sample. Although this method proved to be practical in the clinical laboratory, it was not possible to determine steroid glucuronides directly from diluted urine, due to interfering luminescent compounds. To overcome this problem, we investigated the use of a solid-phase as a separation system since these assays obviate the need for prior purification of the diluted urine (2), and are not significantly affected by background chemiluminescence (2,3).

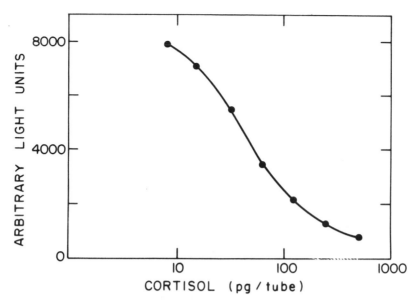

FIG. 2. Representative dose-response curve for cortisol measured by chemiluminescence immunoassay using dextran-coated charcoal as a separation system. Varying amounts of cortisol in 0.1 ml of assay buffer were incubated with anti-cortisol-21-hemisuccinate BSA serum at 1:5,000 dilution (0.1 ml) for 15 min at $37^{\circ}C$ and for 15 min at $4^{\circ}C$. Cortisol-21-hemisuccinate-ABEI conjugate (35 fmol, 0.1 ml) was then added, and the incubation was continued for another 30 min at $4^{\circ}C$. Dextran-coated charcoal was added, and the tubes were processed as described previously (15). The actual light readings recorded on the Luminometer are plotted against log-dose of cortisol.

Solid-phase separation systems

In this method specific antibodies (monoclonal or polyclonal) to steroid glucuronides [estriol-16α-glucuronide (3), estrone-3-glucuronide and pregnanediol-3α-glucuronide (4)] are adsorbed to the walls of Lumacuvettes P polystyrene test tubes. A steroid-glucuronide chemiluminescent marker conjugate and unaltered free steroid glucuronide or diluted urine sample are then allowed to compete for the binding sites of adsorbed IgG. The free fraction is then removed by aspiration and subsequent washing of the tubes with buffer leads to the removal of potentially interfering substances. The light yield of the label bound to adsorbed IgG is then measured by oxidation with a H_2O_2-microperoxidase system at pH 13. Assay curves for pregnanediol-3α-glucuronide and estrone-3-glucuronide were obtained with a range of 15-1,000 pg steroid/ assay tube. Fig. 3 shows a typical dose response curve for estrone-3-glucuronide. As an indication of the sensitivity and reliability of the method oscilloscope tracings of the standard curve for estrone-3-glucuronide are shown in Fig. 4. The solid-

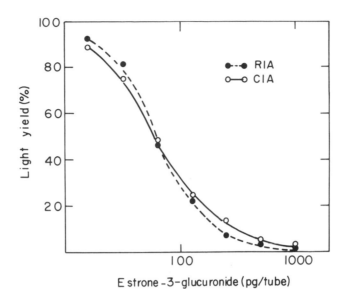

FIG. 3. Representative dose-response curves for estrone-3-glucu-
ronide measured by solid-phase chemiluminescence immunoassay (CIA,
0———0), or solid-phase radioimmunassay (RIA, ●---●). The difference in light yield maximal binding- non-specific binding is taken
as 100% and is plotted against log-dose of estrone-3-glucuronide.

phase chemiluminescence immunoassay for the steroid-glucuronides
(2-4) was validated in terms of specifity, accuracy, sensitivity
and precision. The assay was used to measure estrone-3-glucuron-
ide and pregnanediol-3α-glucuronide in diluted urine samples. Fig.
5 shows daily excretion of estrone-3-glucuronide and pregnanediol-
3α-glucuronide throughout a normal menstrual cycle.

The pattern of the preovulatory **rise** of urinary estrone-3-glu-
curonide excretion, as quantitated by the solid-phase chemiluminescence immunoassay method, was comparable to fluorometric estimates of 24 h urinary total estrogen excretion of six previously
anovulatory women treated with human menopausal gonadotropins (6).

The pregnanediol-3α-glucuronide system was further validated
by comparing assay results with those obtained with the conventional gas liquid chromatographic method (4). The two methods agreed
well (n = 30, r = 0.96). The use of monoclonal antibodies in the
pregnanediol system also facilitates standardization of the assay.

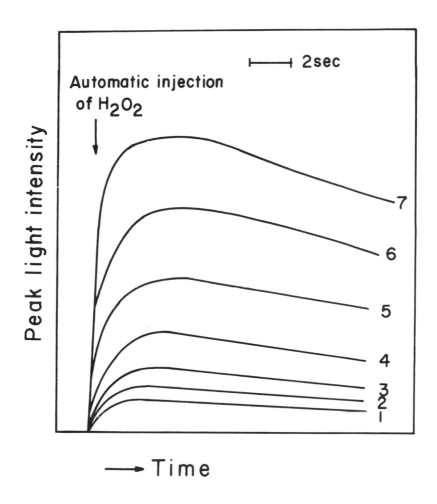

FIG. 4. Oscilloscope tracings of the light signal obtained upon oxidation of estrone-3-glucuronide-ABEI conjugate bound to the antibody-coated tubes with or without addition of estrone-3-glucuronide. Legend: (1) light signal obtained when the enzyme solution only was mixed with the oxidant at pH 13; (2) through (6) light signals obtained when the bound conjugate (50 pg) was oxidized in the presence of varying levels of estrone-3-glucuronide; (2)=100 pg; (3)=50 pg; (4)=25.0 pg; (5)=13 pg; (6)=7 pg; (7) signal due to the oxidation of the conjugate (50 pg) in the antibody-coated tube without the addition of unaltered estrone-3-glucuronide (maximal binding). Scale used on the oscilloscope : speed 2 sec/1.22 cm; sensitivity : 200 mV/1.22 cm.

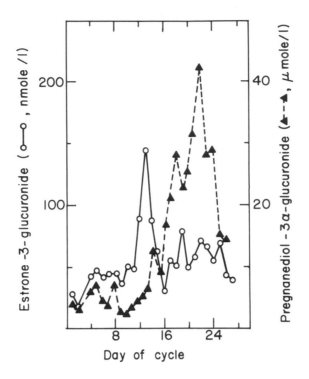

FIG. 5. Daily excretion of estrone-3-glucuronide (0——0) and preg-
nanediol-3α-glucuronide (▲---▲) through a normal menstrual cycle
as measured by solid-phase chemiluminescence immunoassay.

DISCUSSION

In this paper we have discussed several formats of steroid
immunoassays based on monitoring chemiluminescence. These include
"homogeneous" methods not requiring phase separation (8-11), and
heterogeneous methods using dextran-coated charcoal (15-17) or
solid-phase separation systems (2-4). We have shown that in all
these formats the sensitivity achieved was similar to that obtained by conventional RIA methods. However, among these systems, the
solid-phase method was the least affected by background interference problems (2-4). Another added advantage of the solid-phase
system is that there is no need for prior purification of the
diluted urine (2). The steroid-glucuronides are assayed as such,
obviating hydrolysis and extraction steps. The antibody coated
tubes are easy to prepare, can be stored at 4°C for at least six
months, and separation of bound and free hormone is affected by
aspiration.

Better quality control of all types of immunoassay procedures
seems within reach now through the use of monoclonal antibody
preparations (4,5). The monoclonal antibodies used in the development of a solid-phase chemiluminescence immunoassay system for
pregnanediol-3α-glucuronide will always have the same immunochemical specifities since these antibodies can be indefinitely repro-

duced utilizing in vitro (e.g., in tissue culture) or in vivo methods (propagation in ascites fluid of mice).

Although at this stage, recording of the light emission was made manually, the instrumentation required for chemiluminescence immunoassay can probably be produced more cheaply than a scintillation counter. This novel approach to steroid immunoassay appear promising to find a place in clinical laboratories since it offers significant advantages over existing methods in speed, safety and economy.

ACKNOWLEDGEMENTS

The work was supported by grants from the World Health Organization, the Ford Foundation, the Rockefeller Foundation, the G. Schmidt Foundation for Pre-Industrial Research and the U.S.A. Binational Foundation (Jerusalem). J.B. Kim was a visiting scientist from King's College Medical School, London, at the Weizmann Institute of Science. H.R. Lindner is a scholar in residence at the Fogarty International Center of the National Institute of Health. Z. Eshhar is the incumbent of the Recanati Career Development Chair in Cancer Research. We are grateful to Mrs. P. Rubinstein for excellent secretarial assistance, to Mrs. S. Lichter. **Messrs.** N. Zinberg, T. Waks, Mrs. J. Ausler and Mr. A. Almoznino for technical assistance, and to Drs. W. Coulson and P. Samarajeewa, the Courtauld Institute of Biochemistry, The Middlesex Hospital Medical School, London, for the steroid glucu-**ronides** used in this study.

REFERENCES

1. Abraham, G.E., and Garza, R. (1977): Radioimmunoassay of Steroids. In: Handbook of Radioimmunoassay, edited by G.E. Abraham, pp. 591-656, Marcel Debber Inc., New York.

2. Barnard, G., Collins, W.P., Kohen, F. and Lindner, H.R. (1981): A preliminary study of the measurement of urinary pregnane-diol-3α-glucuronide by a solid-phase chemiluminescence immuno-assay. In. Bioluminescence and Chemiluminescence, edited by M.A. DeLuca and W.D. McElroy, pp. 311-317, Academic Press, New York.

3. Barnard, G., Collins, W.P., Kohen, F., and Lindner, H.R. (1981): The measurement of urinary estriol-16α-glucuronide by a solid-phase chemiluminescence immunoassay. J. Steroid Biochem., in press.

4. Eshhar, Z., Kim, J.B., Barnard, G., Collins, W.P., Gilad, S., Lindner, H.R., and **Kohen**, F. (1981): Use of monoclonal antibodies to pregnanediol-3α-glucuronide for the development of a solid-phase chemiluminescence immunoassay. Steroids, in press.

5. Eshhar, Z., Kohen, F. and Lindner, H.R; (1981): Production of monoclonal antibodies to steroid hormones. In: XXIXth Colloquium of Protides of the Biological Fluids, edited by H. Peters, Pergamon Press, Oxford, in press.

6. Kim, J.B., Gilad, S., Kohen, F., Lindner, H.R., Chayen, R., and Peyser, R.M. (1981): Assessment of ovarian function by measurement of urinary steroid glucuronides by a solid-phase chemiluminescence immunoassay method. Israel J. Med. Sci., in press.

7. Kohen, F., Bauminger, S., and Lindner, H.R. (1975). Preparation of antigenic steroid-protein conjugates. In: Steroid Immunoassay, edited by E.H.D. Cameron, S.G. Hillier and K. Griffiths, pp. 11-32, Alpha Omega Publishing Ltd., Cardiff, Wales.

8. Kohen, F., Pazzagli, M., Kim, J.B., Lindner, H.R. and Boguslaski, R.C. (1979): An assay procedure for plasma progesterone based on antibody-enhanced chemiluminescence. FEBS Letts., 104: 201-205.

9. Kohen, F., Kim, J.B., Barnard, G., and Lindner, H.R. (1980): An immunoassay for urinary estriol-16α-glucuronide based on antibody-enhanced chemiluminescence, Steroids, 36: 405-419.

10. Kohen, F., Pazzagli, M., Kim, J.B., and Lindner, H.R. (1980): An immunoassay for plasma cortisol based on chemiluminescence Steroids, 36: 421-438.

11. Kohen, F., Kim, J.B. and Lindner, H.R. (1981): Assay of gonadal steroids based on antibody-enhanced chemiluminescence. In: Bioluminescence and Chemiluminescence, edited by M.A. DeLuca and W.D. McElroy, pp. 357-364, Academic Press, New York.

12. Kohen, F.,Kim, J.B.,Lindner, H.R., and Collins, W.P. (1981): Development of a solid-phase chemiluminescence immunoassay for plasma progesterone, Steroids, in press.

13. Köhler, G. and Milstein, C. (1976): Derivation of specific antibody-producing tissue culture and tumor lines by cell fusion. Eur. J. Immunol., 6: 511-519.

14. Maier, C.L. (1978): Procedure for the assay of pharmacologically, immunologically and biochemically active compounds in biological fluids. United States Patent 4,104,029.

15. Pazzagli, M., Kim, J.B., Messeri, G., Kohen, F., Bolelli, G.F., Tommasi, A., Salerno, R., Moneti, G., and Serio, M. (1981): Luminescent Immunoassay (LIA) of cortisol:1. Synthesis and evaluation of the chemiluminescent labels of cortisol. 2.

Development and validation of the immunoassay monitored by chemiluminescence, J. Steroid Biochem., in press.

16. Pazzagli, M., Kim, J.B., Messeri, G., Martinazzo, G., Kohen, F., Franceschetti, F., Moneti, G., Salerno, R., Tommasi, A. and Serio, M. (1981): Evaluation of different progesterone-isoluminol conjugates for chemiluminescence immunoassay. Clin. Chim. Acta, in press.

17. Pazzagli, M., Kim, J.B., Messeri, G., Martinazzo, G., Kohen, F., Franceschetti, F., Tommasi, A., Salerno, R., and Serio, M. (1981): Luminescent immunoassay (LIA) for progesterone in a heterogeneous system. Clin. Chim. Acta, in press.

18. Pratt, J.J., Woldring, M.G. and Villerius, L. (1978): Chemiluminescence-linked immunoassay. J. Immunol. Methods, 21, 179-186.

19. Schroeder, H.R., Vogelhut, P.O., Carrico, R.J., Boguslaski, R.C. and Buckler, R.T., (1976): Competitive protein binding assay for biotin monitored by chemiluminescence, Anal. Chem., 48: 1933-1937.

20. Schroeder, H.R., Boguslaski, R.C., Carrico, R.J. and Buchler, R.T. (1978): Monitoring specific protein-binding reactions with chemiluminescence. In: Methods in Enzymology, Vol. LVII, edited by M.A. DeLuca, pp. 424-445, Academic Press, New York.

21. Schroeder, H.R. and Yeager, F.M. (1978): Chemiluminescence yields and detection limits of some isoluminol derivatives in various oxidation systems. Anal. Chemistry, 50: 1114-1120.

Luminescent Assays: Perspectives in Endocrinology and Clinical Chemistry, edited by M. Serio and M. Pazzagli, Raven Press, New York © 1982.

The Preparation and Properties of a Chemiluminescent Derivative of 17β-Estradiol

A. Patel, J. S. Woodhead, A. K. Campbell, *R. C. Hart, and *F. McCapra

*Department of Medical Biochemistry, Welsh National School of Medicine, Cardiff CF4 4XN; *School of Molecular Sciences, University of Sussex, Sussex, United Kingdom*

The majority of steroid immunoassays use internally labelled ^{3}H derivatives as radioligands. Though these may have high stability, they have the disadvantages of the inconvenience of β-counting and also relatively low specific activities which may restrict assay sensitivity. ^{125}I can be used to produce labelled steroids with considerably higher specific activities, though their widespread use has been limited by their reduced stability and also by marked differences in antibody affinity between the hapten and the radioligand [1]. Non-isotopic labels, particularly enzymes and fluorescent groups provide high stability, but their sensitivity of detection is rarely better than that of ^{3}H [2,3] as shown in Table 1.

One steroid assay with a requirement for high sensitivity is that of estradiol. Normal plasma levels range from 70 - 260 pmol/l in the follicular phase and from 350 - 1500 pmol/l during the luteal phase of the menstrual cycle. For the measurement of estradiol in the plasma of postmenopausal women (concentrations < 250 pmol/l) and in saliva, the requirement for a high specific activity label cannot be met by currently available techniques.

Chemiluminescent molecules satisfy the criteria for labels in immunoassay [4] in that they can be readily detected with high sensitivity. We have described the successful use of luminol labelled antibodies in immunoassay systems [5].

Chemiluminescence immunoassay of steroids has recently been reported using isoluminol derivatives which have detection limits of

approximately 5×10^{-15} mol (6).   We report here the preparation and
properties of a highly chemiluminescent acridinium ester of 17β-
estradiol, and its potential use as a label for immunoassay.

METHODS

Synthesis of 17β-estradiol acridinium ester

The chemiluminescent derivative was prepared by the esterification
of acridine-9-carboxyl chloride with the 3'-hydroxyl group of estradiol-
17-pyran (prepared from estradiol-3-benzoate, Sigma Chemicals), followed
by the methylation of the nitrogen using methyl fluorosulphonate and
subsequent deprotection of the 17β hydroxyl group (Fig. 1).   It was
then recrystallized from acetone and extensively washed with benzene.

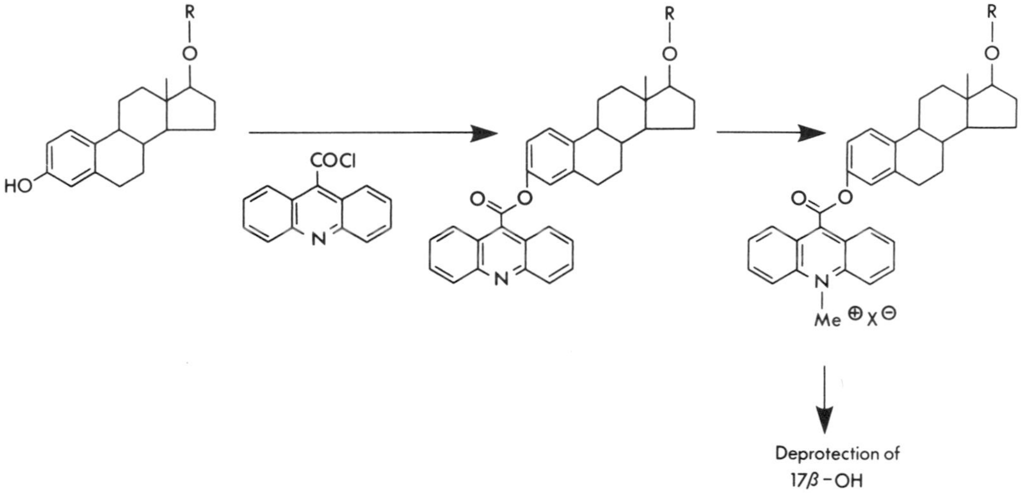

Fig. 1.   Synthesis of 17β-estradiol chemiluminescent derivative.

The conjugate was characterized by thin layer chromatography on
cellulose plates in solvent system of chloroform:95% ethanol (14:1).
The R_f values of the conjugate, estradiol and acridinium-9-carboxylic
acid were 0.89, 0.54 and 0.03 respectively.

Anti-steroid sera

Antisera to estradiol-6-0-carboxylmethyl oxime-BSA conjugate raised in rabbits were generously provided by Dr. G. Read of the Tenovus Institute, Cardiff and Professor W. R. Butt, Birmingham and Midland Hospital for Women, Birmingham, U.K.

Solid phase antiserum

An IgG preparation from one of the antisera obtained from Professor Butt was coupled to a reprecipitated diazonium salt of cellulose (7) and one of the antisera from Dr. Read was obtained already coupled to CNBr-activated cellulose.

Assay procedures

Owing to the high reactivity of acridinium esters all assays were carried out in 0.1 M acetate buffer at pH 5.0. A conventional radio-immunoassay was set up using 25 pg of ^{3}H-estradiol (TRK 322, 85 Ci/mmol, Amersham International, U.K.), an antiserum at a final dilution of 1/8000. Dextran-coated charcoal was used to separate free from bound label after a 2 hr incubation period at 25°C.

The chemiluminescent immunoassay standard curve was set up using a 1/800 dilution of solid-phase antiserum (coupled to cellulose) in a competitive binding system. Separation of the free label after 2 hr incubation at 25°C was achieved by centrifugation of the solid phase, and the luminescence of the free label was measured in an aliquot of the supernatant.

Light measurements

The chemiluminescent derivative is oxidized in the presence of alkaline peroxide to produce excited N-methyl acridone (NMA) and 17β-estradiol. The subsequent deexcitation of the NMA leads to the production of light (Fig. 2).

500 µl of the buffer containing the chemiluminescent derivative was aliquoted into a 3 ml plastic tube and placed in front of a photo-multiplier tube. The derivative was then oxidized by the injection of

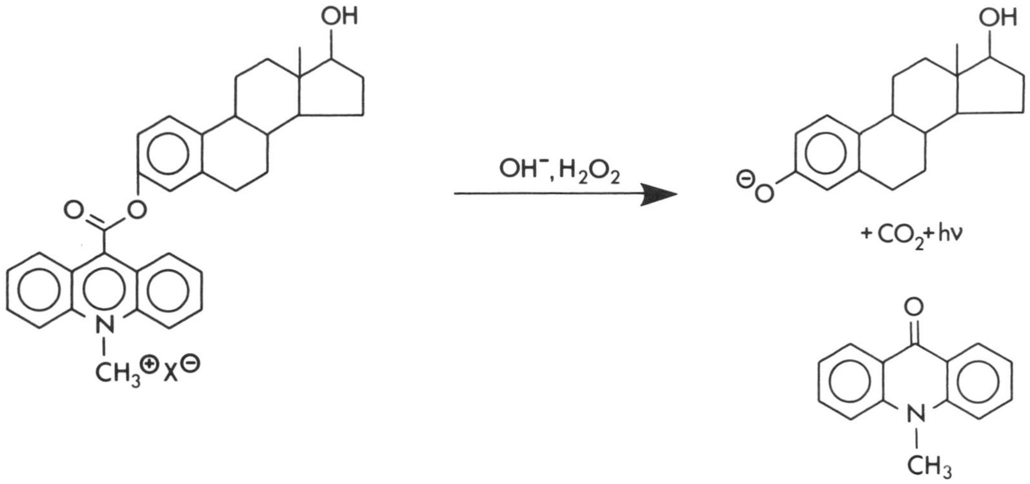

Fig. 2.   Light yielding reaction of 17β-estradiol chemiluminescent
           derivative.

0.8 ml of 0.05% H_2O_2 in 0.5 M NaOH using an automatic injector.   The
light emitted was measured by integrating total counts over a 10 s
period, using a custom-built photon counter (4).

RESULTS

Light-yield of estradiol-acridinium derivative

Under optimized conditions, the light emitted by the chemiluminescent derivative, increased linearly with the amount of the
derivative.   The lower limit of detection (2 SD above buffer blank)
was 2×10^{-17} mol.   The luminescence activity was calculated to be
6.8×10^{18} luminescence counts/mol of the derivative which is comparable
to other acridinium esters which have been studied.

One hundred fmol of the labelled estradiol produced 400,000 luminescent counts in 10 s as compared with an activity of 2,000 scintil-

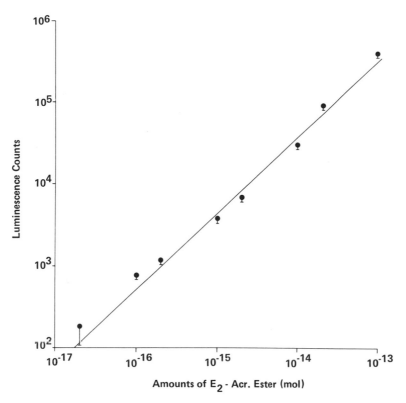

Fig. 3.   Relationship between concentration of chemiluminescent
           derivative (abscissa) and total luminescence (ordinate).

lation counts per minute obtained from an identical quantity of ^{3}H-label.
Because of the high reactivity of acridinium esters care must be taken
regarding storage to prevent potential loss of activity.   However, when
stored as a solid at room temperature or dissolved in dimethyl sulph-
oxide at -20°C, no deterioration of activity of the derivative was noted
over an eight month period.

Immunoreactivity of the derivative

     The immunoreactivity of this label was assessed in a conventional
radioimmunoassay.   While the antiserum bound the chemiluminescent
derivative, it did so with reduced affinity compared with the free
hapten, which is perhaps not surprising owing to the heterologous antisera used.   It was not due to contamination of the derivative with
unreacted estradiol since the labelled compound ran as a single band on
TLC.   The activity of the label was only one twentieth or less that of

free hapten when tested with the four available heterologous antisera.

Antibody dilution curves were set up using equal amounts of either ^{3}H-label or the chemiluminescent label with the solid phase antiserum (cellulose bound). Figure 4 shows the effect of the reduced affinity of the chemiluminescent label on binding. The antibody concentration required for binding 50% of the chemiluminescent label was 8-fold higher than needed to bind an identical quantity of ^{3}H-label.

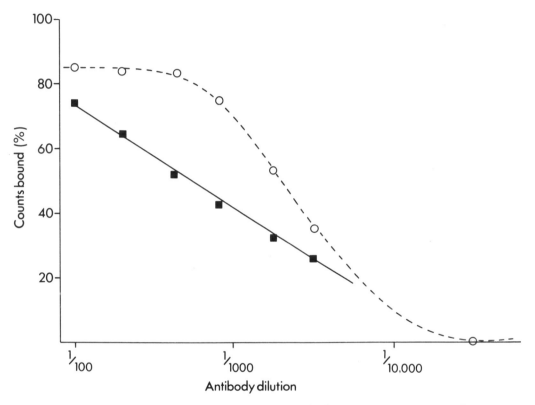

Fig. 4. Antibody dilution curve using solid phase antiserum and (a) ^{3}H-label (o----o) and (b) chemiluminescent label (■——■).

Owing to this reduced affinity, the standard curve obtained with the chemiluminescent label was relatively insensitive and ranged from 0.5 pmol (136 pg) to 500 pmol (1.36 ng) of estradiol per tube (Fig. 5).

DISCUSSION

In recent years a number of chemiluminescent labelled antibodies (5) and steroids (6) have been described for immunoassay purposes based

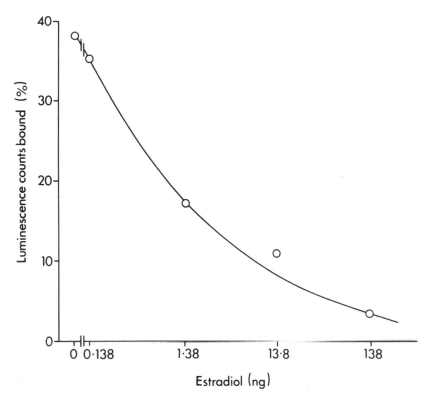

Fig. 5.   17β-estradiol chemiluminescent immunoassay standard curve.

on luminol and its isomers.   Acridinium esters are a group of highly luminescent organic molecules (8) which oxidise readily under mild conditions, with highly reproducible levels of quantitation.   Moreover, the high signal to noise ratio obtained with these derivatives under appropriate conditions enables them to be detected with a high degree of sensitivity.   We have described the preparation of an acridinium ester of 17β-estradiol with a detection limit for the label close to ^{125}I, as shown in Table 1.

Even though high affinity antisera are available for many steroids the sensitivity of assays has been limited by the relatively low specific activity of labels such as ^{3}H and enzymes.

We have prepared a chemiluminescent molecule of estradiol from a non-chemiluminescent precursor which has the quantum yield of the native acridinium ester.   Clearly, the usefulness of this derivative is

Table 1.   Steroid labels used in immunoassay.

Label	Approximate detection limit of label (mol)	Standard curve range
^{3}H	5×10^{-15}	20 - 400 fmol
^{125}I	5×10^{-17}	70 - 3500 fmol
Fluorescent	1×10^{-15}	20 - 400 pmol
Enzyme	6×10^{-16}	10 - 240 fmol
Chemiluminescent: (a) iso-luminol derivatives	5×10^{-15}	25 - 250 fmol
(b) acridinium esters	2×10^{-17}	---

limited by its reduced reactivity with antibodies.   This is not
surprising since the derivative is conjugated through the 3' hydroxyl
group and the antibodies raised against conjugates of 6-0-carboxymethyl
oxime, i.e. a heterologue system.   At present, we are exploring the
use of antisera raised to other conjugates and also the preparation of
alternative labelled derivatives which will yield a more sensitive assay
for estradiol.

We believe that the combination of stability and speed of detection
together with high sensitivity of detection will make chemiluminescent
molecules suitable labels for future immunoassays.

Acknowledgements

This work has been supported by grants from the Department of
Health and Social Security and the Science and Medical Research
Councils.

References

1.   Hunter, W.M., Nars, P.W. and Rutherford, F.J., Proceedings of the
     Fifth Tenovus Workshop Eds. Cameron, E.H.D. et al   Alpha Omega,
     Cardiff. pp 141 - 152 (1975)

2.   Exley, D. and Aruknesha, R., FEBS letters, 91, 162 - 165 (1978)

3.   Dandliker, W.B., Hicks, A.N., Levison, S.A. and Brown, R.J., Res.
     Comm. Chem. Path. Pharm., 18, 147 - 156 (1977)

4. Campbell, A.K. and Simpson, J.S.A., Techniques in Metabolic
    Research, B213, 1 - 56 (1979)

5. Simpson, J.S.A., Campbell, A.K., Ryall, M.E.T. and Woodhead, J.S.,
    Nature 279, 646 - 647 (1979)

6. Kohen, F., Kim, J.B., Barnard, G. and Lindner, H.R., Steroids, 36,
    406 - 420 (1980)

7. Gurevich, A.E., Kuzovleva, O.B. and Lumonova, A.E., Biokhimiya, 26,
    803 (1961)

8. McCapra, F., Tutt, D.E. and Topping, R.M., British Patent No.
    1,461,877 (1977)

Luminescent Assays: Perspectives in Endocrinology and Clinical Chemistry, edited by M. Serio and M. Pazzagli, Raven Press, New York © 1982.

Homogeneous Luminescent Immunoassay for Progesterone: A Study on the Antibody-Enhanced Chemiluminescence

M. Pazzagli, *G. F. Bolelli, **G. Messeri, †G. Martinazzo, A. Tommasi, R. Salerno, and ††M. Serio

*Endocrinology Unit, University of Florence, Florence; *Physiopathology of Reproduction Service, University of Bologna, Bologna; **Clinical Chemistry Laboratory, Careggi, Florence; †Laboratory Research Biodata, Rome; ††Chair of Endocrinology, University of Sassari, Sassari, Italy*

In the last few years, several Luminescent immunoassay (LIA) methods for steroids have been described (1–6). Some of them did not require a phase separation step and were therefore homogeneous (1–4). In homogeneous LIA the CL tracer improves the light yield when it is bound to the antibody. This modification has been defined as the "antibody enhanced CL effect".

The binding between antigen and antibody and the light enhancement can be prevented in a dose–related relationship by the addition of native hormone to the reaction mixture. In Fig.1 an example of a dose response curve for progesterone in homogeneous phase is reported.

Using this approach, homogeneous LIA methods for progesterone (1), cortisol (2) and E_3-glucuronide have been described and applied to the measurement of hormones in biological samples with satisfactory reliability. Homogeneous LIA allow a full automation of the procedure; however they are affected by interfering factors coming from biological samples and the pH of the reaction mixture must be lower than 8.6. Finally, several types of antibody-induced effects on the light emission of label have been observed (see Kohen et al in this volume and Ref.4) and in some cases the enhancement value was not sufficiently high to allow the development of homogeneous LIA. In this paper some preliminary studies on the antibody-enhanced CL phenomenon in progesterone immunoassay are reported.

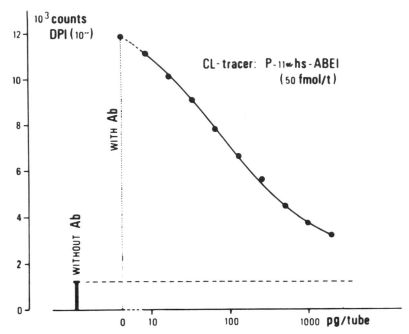

Fig.1 Dose-response curve for progesterone developed in an homogeneous phase. Without antibody: light emission (DF at 10 sec) of 50 fmol/tube of Prog-HS-ABEI. With Ab: light emission of the same amount of steroid but in the presence of a suitable amount anti Prog.-HS-BSA serum. The curve represents the dose-response relationship of the enhancement when different amount of cold progesterone are added to the reaction mixture.

MATERIALS AND METHODS

Progesterone-CL conjugates used in this study have been synthesized, purified and characterized by mass spectra and UV spectra according to Ref.5 and 6 (see also Messeri et al in this volume) The synthesized compounds have been listed in Tab.1. Antisera anti-progesterone 11alfa-hemisuccinate-BSA have been obtained in rabbits and evaluated in terms of titre and affinity constant (Ka) as reported in Tab.2.

Measurements of light emission have been performed with a Luminometer Berthold Biolumat LB 9500 (Wildbad,FRG)(see Ref. 5 for definitions of light measurements).

All other reagents (buffers, oxidation system, ecc.) have been used as previously described (5,6).

RESULTS

Measurements of CL reaction in homogeneous LIA.

Tab.1 Progesterone CL labelled conjugates with different
      structure of CL label or of the bridge(6).

HOMOLOGOUS BRIDGE

Progesterone-11alfa-hemisuccinate-AEI	P-11HS-AEI
" " " -AEEI	P-11HS-AEEI
" " " -ABI	P-11HS-ABI
" " " -ABEI	P-11HS-ABEI
" " " -AHEI	P-11HS-AHEI

HETEROLOGOUS BRIDGE

| Progesterone-11alfa-hemiphtalate-ABEI | P-11HS-ABEI |

In Fig.2 several CL reactions have been reported; reaction
a) was the light yield of 20 fmol/tube of P-11HS-ABEI. 100
fmol/tube produced the reaction b)(a five fold increment
measuring TLP as well as PLI or DPI). It is evident that under
these experimental conditions any parameter can be efficiently
used for monitoring the increment in light emission. This is
the case of CL reactions for LIA measurement in heterogeneous
system.

On the other hand the addition of suitable amount of the
specific antibody to the reaction a) (left side of Fig.2)
produced an enhancement in light yield of about 6 fold as
measured by TLP. This enhancement, however was just 2 fold
when PLI has been measured and 10 fold when DPI has been used.
On the basis of these experiments we can conclude that the

Tab.2 Titre and Ka value of the antisera anti Progesterone-
      HS-BSA employed in this study.[+]

ANTISERA ANTI-PROGESTERONE-11alfa-HEMISUCCINATE-BSA

1) C 89   Titre: 1:16.000
                  Ka   : 7.54×10^9 L/M

2) CU 113   Bleeding date   Titre   Ka

                  a) nov.22, 1979   1:6.200 3×10^9
                     may 20, 1980   BOOSTER INJ.
                  b) may 30, 1980   1:16.500 5×10^9
                  c) jun.20, 1980   1:15.000 5×10^9
                  d) jul.28, 1980   1:7.000 4×10^9

[+] Titre and Ka value of the antisera have been
    determined using tritiated progesterone (and
    the Scatchard's Plot method).

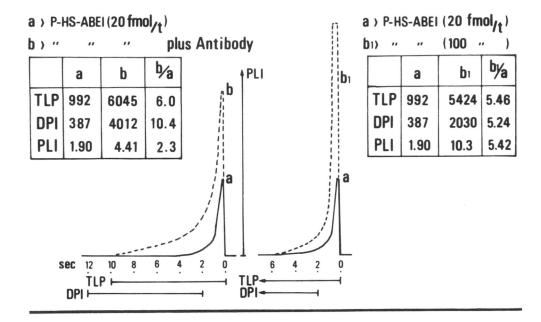

Fig.2 Oscilloscope tracings and readings on the luminometer
display of some CL reactions. TLP= total light production,
DPI= decay portion integration, PLI= peak light intensity.
    On the right side of the figure, two different CL
reaction are reported where b_1 has been obtained increasing
the amount of the CL conjugate (5 fold).
    On the left side of the figure, two different reactions
are reported where b has been obtained by adding to the
reaction mixture an aliquot of antiserum anti-P-11HS-BSA.
Reaction conditions are as reported in Ref.5 .

light enhancement is not only a simple quantitative effect
but also a qualitative modification of light emission. In
other words, the kinetics of light emission may be affected
by the addition of the antibody. Therefore the choice of a
suitable parameter for light measurement is mandatory to
obtain the best results in homogeneous LIA.

The chemical structure of the CL-labelled progesterone on the antibody enhanced chemiluminescence effect

    Several progesterone CL conjugates have been investigated.
The chemical structure of the CL label and of the bridge
between the label and the steroid molecule has been variously
modified (see Tab.1);the CL conjugates have been studied in
the presence or absence of anti-Progesterone-11HS-BSA serum.
    The use of a heterologous bridge (hemiphtalate instead of

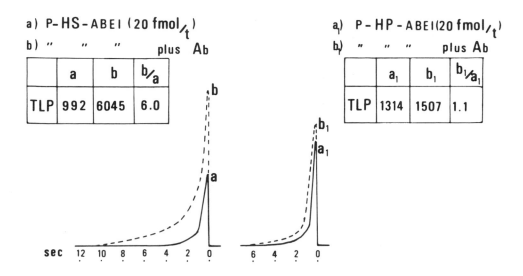

Fig.3 Effect of modifications on the chemical structure of the bridge between the steroid and the CL label on the antibody enhanced chemiluminescence. Two different conjugates of Progesterone (hemisuccinate and hemiphtalate) have been oxidized in the absence or in the presence of antiserum anti–P–11HS–BSA. For experimental conditions see Fig.2.

hemisuccinate) provoked a suitable enhancement (see Fig.4).

However the enhancement values of the same conjugate have been found consistently different, depending on the paramater used for the light measurement. Moreover differences between the conjugates have been found even considering the same parameter for light measurement (see Fig.4,5).

Since the homologous-bridge conjugate produced suitable enhancement, we studied the slope and range of dose response curves which could be obtained using different conjugates.

The results are reported in Fig.6. Significant differences in dose-response curves have been observed.

In conclusion, the chemical structure of the Progesterone CL conjugate seems to play an important role on the enhancement. Modifications of the chemical structure of the bridge as well as of the the amino residues of the isoluminol derivative can produce significant differences on the reaction kinetics, on the enhancement values and finally on the dose response curves.

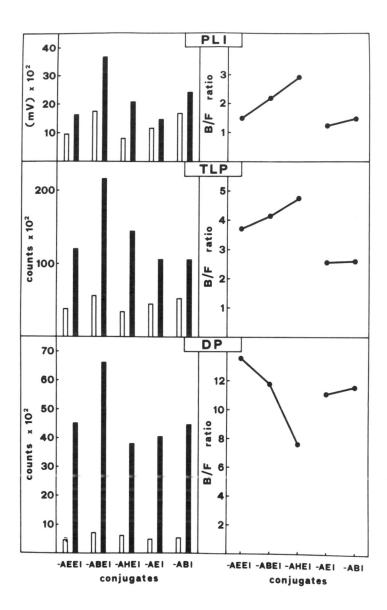

Fig.4 On the left PLI, TLP and DP values are reported
   as produced by different homologous-bridge conjugates in
   in presence (black bars) and in absence (white bars) of
   anti-progesterone-11HS-BSA serum. 50 fmol/tube of each
   conjugate have been used through all the experiments.
      On the right this phenomenon has been expressed in
   terms of ratio between antibody enhanced luminescence and
   basal light emission.

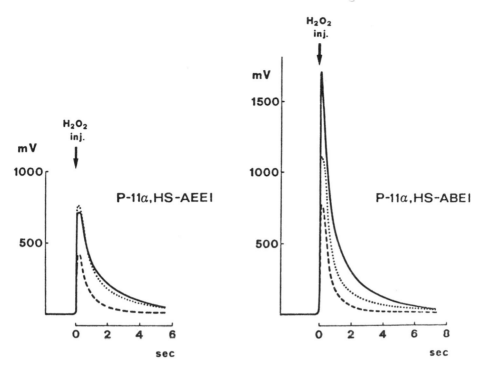

Fig.5 Oscilloscope tracings of CL reactions for homogeneous
    LIA obtained using two different CL-labelled progesterone
    conjugates.
    (- - - -) Oxidation reaction of 50 fmol/tube of
            conjugate in the absence of the antibody
    (—————) Oxidation reaction of 50 fmol/tube of
            conjugate in the presence of a fixed amount of
            anti-Progesterone-11HS-BSA serum.
    (.......) Effect of 1000 pg/tube addition of cold
            progesterone to the reaction mixture.

The role of the antibody on the antibody enhanced chemiluminescence effect

   Experiments have been carried out using the same CL tracer
reacting with antisera from different bleedings or antisera
from different animals (see Tab.2).
   Antisera have been evaluated in terms of maximum
enhancement in titration curves using the same CL labelled
progesterone (P-11HS-ABEI). The results are reported in
Fig.7. Significant differences have been observed in
relation to the antibody used for the reaction. Therefore
the antibody can produce significant modification on the
enhancement phenomenon.

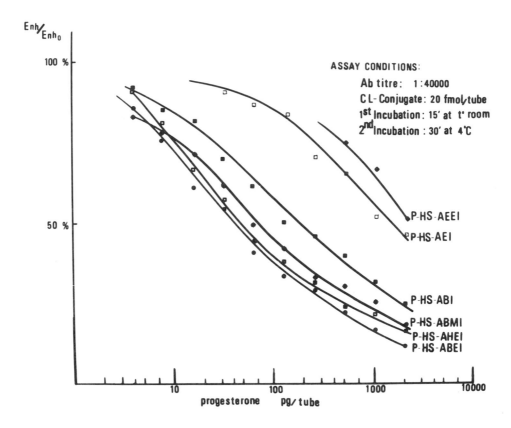

Fig.6 Dose-response curves for progesterone in an homo-
       geneous system as obtained using different CL-labelled
       Progesterone conjugates.

DISCUSSION

Homogeneous LIA methods for steroids are attractive
procedures because they allow a full automation of the
assay. However at this moment they have some disadvantages
mainly due to an incomplete knowledge of the mechanism of
the antibody-enhanced chemiluminescence.

In this paper we have examined several factors that
could be involved in the enhancement phenomenon. All the
investigated parameter (method of light measurement, the
chemical structure of the tracer, the antibody) have been
found able to affect the enhancement value. Consequently it
seems that the development of optimal homogeneous LIA
will   be possible only when well standardized reagent will
be available.

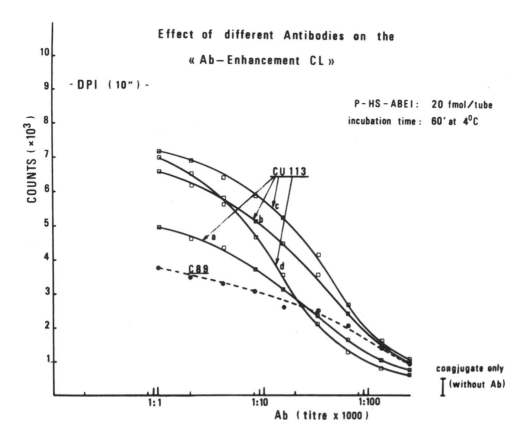

Fig.7 Titration curves obtained using different antibodies
    as reported in Tab.2

ACKNOWLEDGEMENTS

This work was supported by a Grant from the University of
Florence.

REFERENCES

1) Kohen,F.,Pazzagli,M.,Kim,J.B.,Lindner,H.R. and Bogulaski,
   R.C. (1979): FEBS Letts., 14, 201-205.
2) Kohen,F.,Pazzagli,M.,KimJ.B.,H.R. (1980): Steroids, 36,
   421-435.
3) Kohen,F.,Kim,J.B.,Barnard,G.,Lindner,H.R.(1980):Steroids
   36,405-420.
4) Kohen,F.,Kim,J.B.,Lindner,H.R. (1981): in Bioluminescence
   and Chemiluminescence, edited by M.A. De Luca and W.D.
   McElroy, pp. 357-364. Academic Press,New York.
5) Pazzagli,M.,Kim,J.B.,Messeri,G.,Martinazzo,G.,Kohen,F.,
   Franceschetti,F.,Moneti,G.,Salerno,R.,Tommasi,A.and
   Serio,M. (1981): J.Steroid Biochem., in press.

6) Pazzagli,M.;Kim,J.B.,Messeri,G.,Kohen,F.,Bolelli,G.F.,
   Tommasi,A.,Salerno,R.,Moneti,G,and Serio,M. (1981):
   Clin.Chim.Acta, in press.
7) Schroeder,H.R., Voghelhut,P.O.,Carrico,R.J.,Bogulaski,
   R.C.and Buckler,R.T. (1976): Anal. Chem., 48, 1933-1937.

Luminescent Assays: Perspectives in Endocrinology and Clinical Chemistry, edited by M. Serio and M. Pazzagli, Raven Press, New York © 1982.

Measurement of Plasma Progesterone by a Solid-Phase Chemiluminescence Immunoassay Method

*J. B. Kim, F. Kohen, H. R. Lindner, and *W. P. Collins

*Department of Hormone Research, The Weizmann Institute of Science, Rehovot 76100, Israel; *Department of Obstetrics and Gynaecology, King's College Hospital Medical School, London SE5 8RX, Great Britain*

Ovarian luteal function can be assessed by determination of plasma progesterone, and radioimmunoassay (RIA) is widely used for this purpose because of its high sensitivity and specificity. However, RIA may pose problems related to the use of an isotopically labelled antigen, the disposal of radioactive waste and the high cost of the equipment required. Immunoassays based on monitoring chemiluminescence do not have these drawbacks and recent studies using biotin (11) or steroid (5-8) models suggest that this approach may afford a feasible alternative to radioimmunoassay.

In continuation of our attempts to develop a practical immunoassay for plasma progesterone based on monitoring chemiluminescence we investigated the use of a solid phase separation method for the development of the assay. In the method described here a γ-immunoglobulin fraction to progesterone-11α-hemisuccinate bovine serum albumin is adsorbed to the walls of polystyrene test tubes. A chemiluminescent marker conjugate of progesterone and unaltered free steroid are then allowed to compete for the binding sites of adsorbed IgG. The free fraction is removed by aspiration and subsequent washing of the tubes with buffer leads to the removal of potentially interfering substances. The label bound to adsorbed IgG is then measured using chemiluminescence as an end point. The results of an immunoassay for plasma progesterone based on a solid-phase separation system are reported here.

MATERIALS AND METHODS

11α-Hydroxy-4-pregnene-3,20-dione 11-hemisuccinate was linked covalently to 6[N-(4-aminobutyl)-N-ethyl]-amino-2,3-dihydrophthalazine-1,4-dione (ABEI) (12) to yield progesterone-ABEI conjugate (Fig. 1), essentially as previously described (8-10).

Antiserum to progesterone was raised in rabbits, using a progesterone-11-hemisuccinate-bovine serum albumin conjugate as the immunogen (4). Anti-progesterone IgG fraction was prepared and characterized as previously described (5). All other reagents and assay procedures were as previously described (9). Light emission was measured with a Luminometer Model 2080 (Lumac Systems, Basel).

Collection of plasma. Blood (10 ml) was withdrawn by venepuncture and collected in glass tubes containing 0.1 ml of heparin. Plasma was separated by centrifugation, transferred to glass tubes and stored at -20°C until analysis.

Sample preparation. Each plasma sample (0.5 ml) was extracted with 10 ml of redistilled petroleum ether. The organic extract was dried under a stream of nitrogen and assay buffer (1 ml) was added to the dried residue. A portion (0.5 ml) of this solution was used for the chemiluminescence immunoassay. The remainder was used for radioimmunoassay when comparison of the two methods was made.

Antibody-coated tubes. Lumacuvette Polystyrene P test tubes (Lumac Systems, Basel) were coated with anti-progesterone IgG as previously described (9).

Immunoassay procedure. Dose response curves were established at the beginning and end of the assay. The unknown samples were run in duplicate and at two different dilutions. The assay was assembled as shown below (Table 1).

Calculations. The decrease in light yield induced by standards or samples is expressed as a percentage of the difference between maximal binding - non-specific binding. From a plot of these percentages the progesterone concentration of unknown sample is read, and the plasma progesterone concentration is calculated.

RESULTS

A chemiluminescence immunoassay for progesterone. Using the progesterone-ABEI conjugate (Fig. 1) and conditions described in Legend to Fig. 2, an assay curve for progesterone was obtained with a linear segment between 15-1000 pg progesterone/tube.

Reliability of the chemiluminescence immunoassay and application to biological material. The recovery of tritiated progesterone added to plasma by the extraction procedure described in the Methods section was 94.2%+2.7 S.D. (n=20).

The specificity of the immunoassay using anti-progesterone IgG by the solid-phase chemiluminescence immunoassay was similar to that observed by radioimmunoassay using the same antiserum. Light emission was unaffected by addition of cortisol or estradiol. Minor cross-reaction was observed with 17α-hydroxyprogesterone (0.5%), 11β-hydroxyprogesterone (12%) and 11α-hydroxyprogesterone (23%). Varying amounts of progesterone were added to a pool of male plasma (0.4-10 ng/ml), and the samples were then assayed by chemiluminescence immunoassay. Satisfactory correlation was obtained between amount added and amount recovered (r=0.98; n=12).

The sensitivity of the assay was comparable to that obtained in RIA

TABLE 1

LAY-OUT OF THE SOLID PHASE CHEMILUMINESCENCE IMMUNOASSAY

Type of tube used	Regular Lumacuvette		Antibody-coated Lumacuvette		
	Designation of Tube				
	(A)	(B)	(C)	(D)	(E)
Reagent Added	Enzyme/ Oxidant Blank	Total Counts	Non-specific Blank	Maximal Binding	Sample or Standard
Buffer	0.2 ml	0.1 ml	0.1 ml	0.2 ml	-
Marker Conjugate	-	0.1 ml	0.1 ml	0.1 ml	0.1 ml
Sample or Standard	-	-	-	-	0.2 ml

1. Incubate 1 to 2 hr at room temperature.
2. Aspirate and wash twice, tubes designated (C), (D) and (E).

NaOH (1N)	0.1 ml	0.1 ml	0.1 ml	0.1 ml	0.1 ml
Buffer	-	-	0.2 ml	0.2 ml	0.2 ml

Incubate all tubes at room temperature for 30 min. Add enzyme solution (0.1 ml) to all the tubes, inject oxidant (0.1 ml) to each tube in the dark and measure light emission.

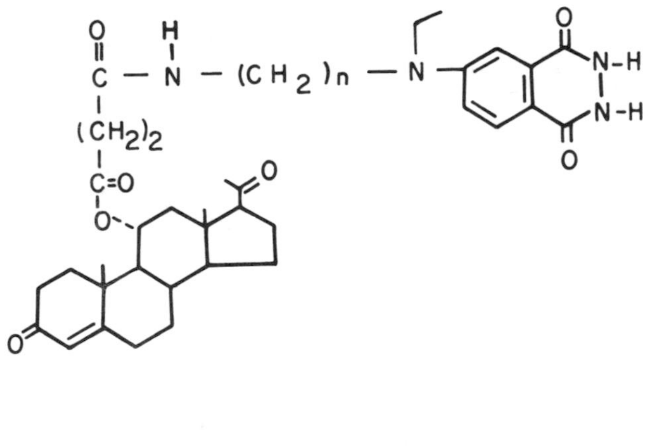

FIG. 1. The proposed structure of progesterone-ABEI conjugate; n=4.

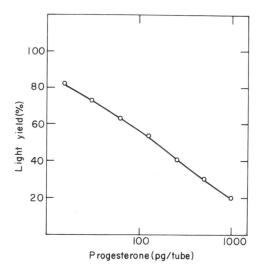

FIG. 2. A dose-response curve for progesterone measured by solid-phase chemiluminescence immunoassay. Varying amounts of progesterone were incubated with progesterone-ABEI conjugate (25 pg) in Lumacuvettes coated with anti-progesterone-IgG at 1:1000 dilution and processed as described in Table 1. The difference in light yield maximal binding-non-specific binding is taken at 100% and is plotted against log-dose of progesterone.

procedures. The least amount of progesterone that could be distinguished from zero (p<0.05) was 10 pg/tube.

The reproducibility of the assay was evaluated by performing replicate determinations of the same sample in one assay and in four different assays. The coefficient of variation (C.V.) of the results of duplicate determinations from their means was estimated according to (1). On 20 replicate determinations performed in the same assay, the mean progesterone content of a luteal phase plasma was 9.4+0.7 ng/ml and the coefficient of variation was 7.4%. In three duplicate determinations in four different assays the coefficient of variation was 9.8%.

Progesterone concentration in human plasma. Plasma samples from normally ovulating women and from anovulatory women undergoing pergonal treatment were assayed by chemiluminescence immunoassay. The values obtained for plasma progesterone levels in normally menstruating subjects were in accordance with those obtained by established methodologies. Likewise, treatment of six previously anovulatory women with human menopausal gonatropins, followed by human chorionic gonadotropin, led to the expected rise in plasma progesterone level from <1 ng/ml to 6.1-15.3 ng progesterone/ml.

Several samples from non-pregnant women taken at different stages of the menstrual cycle (n=33) were extracted with petroleum ether, and the extracts were assayed for progesterone by radioimmunoassay and by chemiluminescence immunoassay using the same antiserum. Satisfactory correla-

tion of the results was obtained between the two methods, r=0.98;
y=1.06x0.20, where y corresponds to values determined by radioimmunoassay (Fig. 3).

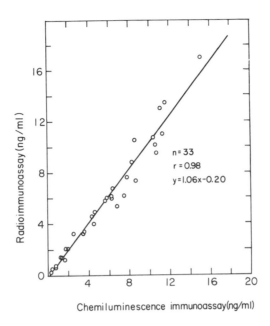

FIG. 3. Comparison of plasma progesterone levels as determined by solid-
phase RIA or solid-phase chemiluminescence immunoassay.

DISCUSSION

The results of this pilot trial of a solid-phase chemiluminescence
based immunoassay for plasma progesterone, combined with similar results
for solid-phase chemiluminescence assay systems for urinary estriol-16α-
glucuronide (2), and for pregnanediol-3α-glucuronide (3), indicate that
this novel approach to steroid immunoassay is sufficiently promising to
warrant more extensive exploration. Potential advantages over RIA could
be the lack of radioactive waste. Unlike homogeneous chemiluminescence
immunoassays (4-8) this method is not affected by background interference
from extracts of samples of biological origin, since potentially interfering luminescent compounds are removed by aspiration after the binding
reaction. Although at this stage, recording of the light emission was
made manually, the lack of a centrifugation step makes the assay readily
amenable to automation.

ACKNOWLEDGEMENTS

This work was supported by grants from the World Health Organization,
the Ford Foundation, the Rockefeller Foundation, the G. Schmidt Foundation for Pre-Industrial Research. H.R. Lindner is a scholar in residence

at the Fogarty International Center of the National Institute of Health. We are grateful to Mrs. R. Levin for excellent secretarial assistance, to Mrs. S. Lichter. Mrs. J. Ausher and Mr. A. Almoznino for technical assistance.

REFERENCES

1. Abraham, G.E., and Garza, R. (1977): In: Handbook of Radioimmunoassay, edited by G.E. Abraham, pp. 591-656. Marcel Deccer Inc., New York.

2. Barnard, G., Collins, W.P., Kohen, F., and Lindner, H.R. (1981): J. Steroid Biochem., in press.

3. Eshhar, Z., Kim, J.B., Barnard, G., Collins, W.P., Gilad, S., Lindner, H.R., and Kohen, F. (1981): Steroids, in press.

4. Kohen, F., Bauminger, S., and Lindner, H.R. (1975): In: Steroid Immunoassay, edited by E.H.D. Cameron, S.G. Hillier, and K. Griffiths, pp. 11-32. Alpha Omego Publishing Ltd., Cardiff, Wales.

5. Kohen, F., Pazzagli, M., Kim, J.B., Lindner, H.R., and Boguslaski,R.C. (1979): FEBS Letts., 104:201-205.

6. Kohen, F., Kim, J.B., Barnard, G., and Lindner, H.R. (1980): Steroids, 36:405-419.

7. Kohen, F., Pazzagli, M., Kim, J.B., and Lindner, H.R. (1980): Steroids, 36:421-438.

8. Kohen, F., Kim, J.B., and Lindner, H.R. (1981): In: Bioluminescence and Chemiluminescence, edited by M.A. DeLuca and W.D. McElroy, pp. 357-364. Academic Press, New York.
9.
Kohen, F., Kim, J.B., Lindner, H.R., and Collins, W.P. (1981): Steroids, in press.

10. Pazzagli, M., Kim, J.B., Messeri, G., Martinazzo, G., Kohen, F., Franceschetti, F., Moneti, G., Salerno, R., Tommasi, A., and Serio, M. (1981): Clin. Chim. Acta, in press.

11. Schroeder, H.R., Vogelhut, P.O., Carrico, R.J., Boguslaski, R.C., and Buckler, R.T. (1976): Anal. Chem., 48:1933-1937.

12. Schroeder, H.R., Boguslaski, R.C., Carrico, R.J., and Buchler, R.T. (1978): In: Methods in Enzymology, Vol. LVII, edited by M.A. DeLuca, pp. 424-445. Academic Press, New York.

*Luminescent Assays: Perspectives in
Endocrinology and Clinical Chemistry*, edited by
M. Serio and M. Pazzagli, Raven Press,
New York © 1982.

Chemiluminescent Tracers for Steroid Measurements

G. Messeri, *G. Martinazzo, **A. Tommasi, †G. Moneti,
**R. Salerno, **M. Pazzagli, ††and M. Serio

*Clinical Chemistry Laboratory, Careggi, Florence; *Laboratory Research Biodata,
Rome; **Endocrinology Unit and †Mass Spectrometry Unit, University of Florence, Florence; ††Chair
of Endocrinology, University of Sassari, Sassari, Italy*

The quantum yield of the chemiluminescent (CL) reaction is one of the most important factors affecting the sensitivity of CL monitored immunoassays and it mainly depends on the oxidation system and the chemical structure of the CL compound.

The aim of the present report has been to investigate the contribution of some CL compounds to the light yield of the reaction. To this purpose a number of isoluminol derivatives have been synthesized (Fig. 1). Such labels have been then covalently linked to various steroids. The light efficiency of labels and conjugates have been finally evaluated.

In order to get standard conditions, the same oxidation system has been used through all the experiments. The H_2O_2-microperoxidase system has been selected because of its widely reported (4) sensitivity and practicability.

Since it is quite difficult to perform absolute light yield measurements, luminol has been used in each series of experiments as a reference compound. Because of its high light efficiency, it has been widely investigated under many oxidation systems by many authors (4) and it appears as an ideal reference compound.

Light output has been reported to be quantified by many ways, and mainly by Peak Light Intensity, Decay Portion Integration and Total Light Production measurements (2).

We have chosen Total Light Production measurement because

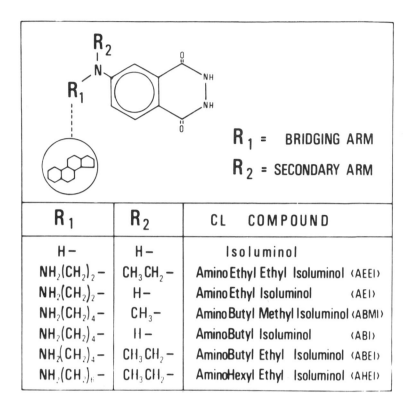

Fig.1   Structure and nomenclature of the synthesized iso-
         luminol derivatives.

 it does not strictly depends on the reaction kinetics, it
appears well representative of the amount of photons emitted
in the course of the entire reaction and well related to
quantum efficiency.
   A further source of inaccuracy,in efficiency evaluation
experiments, is the possibility that a variation of the
reaction conditions causes a shift of the emission wavelenght.
As the phototube sensitivity is wavelenght dependent, a large
shift of emission maximum should affect the total light measurements. The resulting variation could be erroneously attributed to a different quantum efficiency. Therefore, the
constancy of the emission wavelenght has always been checked
when changing the reaction conditions.

                    MATERIAL   AND METHODS

   Chemiluminescent compounds have been synthesised according
to Schroeder et al.(4) and characterized by electron impact
ionisation mass spectrometry (Fig.2).

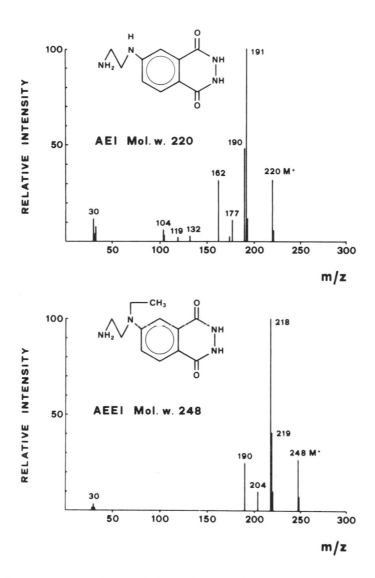

Fig. 2 Mass spectra of two isoluminol derivatives, as
        obtained by the usual electron impact ionisation.

Steroids conjugates (Tab.1) have been prepared as previously described (1,2). Their purity has been checked by
U.V. spectra and bidimensional TLC (3). The compounds identity has been confirmed by mass spectrometry. Because of the
thermal instability of these molecules, field desorption
instead of electron impact ionisation has been used as the
ions producing tecnique (Fig.3).

Tab.1 Synthesis and nomenclature of some CL-labelled
steroids

Steroid Derivative	CL - Label	Conjugate
Cortisol - 21 HS	ABI	C - 21 HS-ABI
	ABEI	C - 21 HS-ABEI
Progesterone - 11 HS	AEI	P - 11 HS-AEI
	AEEI	P - 11 HS-AEEI
	ABI	P - 11 HS-ABI
	ABMI	P - 11 HS-ABMI
	ABEI	P - 11 HS-ABEI
	AHEI	P - 11 HS-AHEI
Testosterone - 3 CMO	ABI	T - 3 CMO-ABI
	ABEI	T - 3 CMO-ABEI
	AEEI	T - 3 CMO-AEEI
Testosterone - 17 HS	ABI	T - 17 HS-ABI
	ABEI	T - 17 HS-ABEI
	AEEI	T - 17 HS-AEEI
Estradiol - 6 CMO	ABEI	E_2 - 6 CMO-ABEI
Estradiol - 17 HS	ABEI	E_2 - 17 HS-ABEI

The chemiluminescent reaction has been carried out under
the previously described conditions (2). Light measurements
have been performed with a Biolumat Berthold LB 9500 by integrating the light output over a 60 sec period. Such a time
has been found long enough to measure at least 90% of the
light emitted in the course of the slowest reaction.

RESULTS

The light efficiency evaluation of synthesized compounds,
as carried on under the above stated conditions, yielded the
following results:
1) Light efficiency of isoluminol derivatives is pH dependent
2) The amino group of isoluminol plays a main role in determining the molecule light yield, and particulary:
   a) the introduction of one alkyl group markly increases
      the light efficiency (Tab.2), but the pH value yielding
      the highest emission is constricted in a small range,
      around 11 (Fig.4)

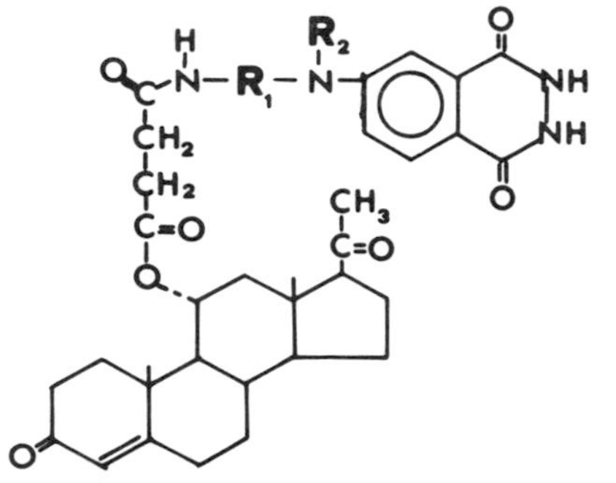

CONJUGATE	R_1	R_2	M.W. a.u.	M^+	$(M+H)^+$	$(M+H)_2^{+\cdot}$	$(M+N_a)$
P-11α-HS-AEI	$(CH_2)_2$	-H	632	632	633		655
P-11α-HS-AEEI	$(CH_2)_2$	-CH$_2$CH$_3$	660	660	661		683
P-11α-HS-ABI	$(CH_2)_4$	-H	660	660	661		683
P 11α-HS-ABEI	$(CH_2)_4$	-CH$_2$CH$_3$	688	688	689		711
P 11α-HS-AHEI	$(CH_2)_6$	-CH$_2$CH$_3$	716	716	717		739
P 11α-HS-ABMI	$(CH_2)_4$	-CH$_3$	674		675		697

Fig.3 Mass spectra results from steroid-conjugates, as
       obtained by the field desorption technique

b) the introduction of two alkyl groups not only produces
   a large increase of quantum efficiency (Tab.3) but the
   optimal pH range get wider (Fig.4, right).

Tab.2 Detection limits of some chemiluminescent labels

CL Label	Optimal pH range	Detection limit (fmoles/tube)
Luminol	10 - 11	0.2
Isoluminol	10 - 11	1.5
AEI	10 - 11	0.5
AEEI	10 - 13	0.1
ABI	10 - 11	1.0
ABMI	10 - 13	0.3
ABEI	10 - 13	0.2
AHEI	10 - 13	0.5

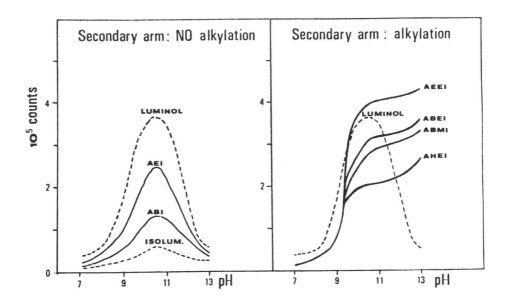

Fig.4   Effect on light emission of 100 fmoles/tube of some
        CL labels.

3) The conjugation of isoluminol derivatives to steroid hemi-
   succinates do not affect either the quantum yield of the
   label or the pH dependence, as regards both mono and di-
   alkylated molecules.
4) The conjugation to steroid carboxy-methyl-oxyme saves the
   pH dependence but results a three-four fold decrease in
   terms of light efficiency. This decrement following the
   conjugation step may be caused by the position of the
   bridge to the steroid molecule, by the chemical structure
   of the bridge itself or both. This phenomena has already
   been reported for other compounds and proves that the
   conjugate efficiency depends not only on the label light
   efficiency but on the steroid chemical structure too.

CONCLUSIONS

   It has been largely claimed that CL tracers are quite
stable, mostly when compared to radioisotopic tracers.There
is no evidence about their toxicity and their use does not
requires any licence. CL tracers can be detected rapidly at
fmole level and their sensitivity is comparable to that we
can obtain by radioactivity.
   It is worth remembering, talking about sensitivity, that
each mplecule of the CL tracer is labelled, while the radioisotopic tracer is a mixture of cold and labelled molecules.

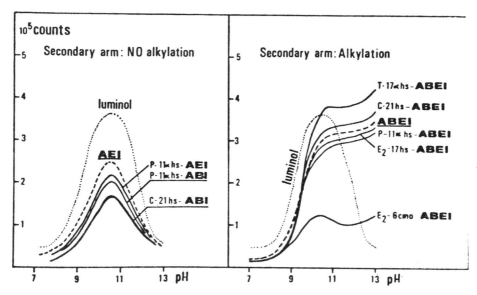

Fig.5 Effect of pH on light emission of 100 fmoles/tube of some CL-labelled steroids.

As regards our report. some relations have been established between the well known chemical structure of some compounds and their CL efficiency. This approach is however of poor value when dealing about the efficiency of a tracer suitable for homogeneous immunoassay. In this case the efficiency is related to the light enhancement which follows the antibody binding and depends on both the CL compound and the antiserum used.

Tab. 3   Detection limits of some CL-labelled steroids

CL-Compound	Detection Limit (fmols/tube)
AEEI	0.1
P-11 HS-AEEI	0.2
T-17 HS-AEEI	0.1
T-3 CMO-AEEI	0.7
ABEI	0.2
P-11 HS-ABEI	0.2
C-21 HS-ABEI	0.2
T-17 HS-ABEI	0.1
E_2-17 HS-ABEI	0.2
T-3 CMO-ABEI	0.7
E_2-6 CMO-ABEI	0.5

However, the exact knowledge of the chemical structure of the tracer and the possibility of modifying such a structure to improve the assay features appears as one of the most interesting aspect of the CL tracers.

REFERENCES

1) Kohen,F., Pazzagli,M., Kim,J.B., Lindner,H.R.and Bogulaski R.C. (1979): FEBS Letters, 104, 201-205.

2) Pazzagli,M., Kim,J.B., Messeri,G., Martinazzo,G., Kohen, F., Franceschetti,F., Moneti, G., Salerno,R., Tommasi,A. and Serio,M. (1981): J.Steroid Biochem. , in press

3) Pazzagli,M., Kim,J.B., Messeri,G., Kohen,F., Bolelli,G.F., Tommasi,A., Salerno,R., Moneti,G. and Serio,M. (1981): Clin.Chim.Acta,in press

4) Schroeder,H.R.and Yeager,F.M. (1978): Anal.Chem.,50, 1114 -1120

5) Schroeder,H.R., Voghelhut,P.O.,Carrico,R.J.,Bogulaski, R. C. and Buckler,R.T. (1976): Anal.Chem., 48, 1933-1937.

*Luminescent Assays: Perspectives in
Endocrinology and Clinical Chemistry*, edited by
M. Serio and M. Pazzagli, Raven Press,
New York © 1982.

Compartmentalisation and Defenses Against Active Oxygens in Intact Cells and Organelles as Investigated with Site Specific, Chemiluminescent Probes

Richard D. Lippman

*Department of Medical Cell Biology, University of Uppsala, Uppsala, Sweden S-75123 and
Division of Physical Chemistry, Royal Institute of Technology,
S-10044 Stockholm, Sweden*

In the study of cellular energy and metabolism, the superoxide anion radical ($O_2^-\bullet$) and its active-oxygen biproducts ($\bullet OH$, H_2O_2, $^1O_2$) have attracted great interest in recent years (4,12). A suitable method of detection inside <u>intact</u> cells and organelles has been lacking. The use of site-specific chemiluminescent probes for the measurement of $O_2^-\bullet$ and $\bullet OH$ in metabolically-active cells and organelles circumvents many earlier experimental difficulties (5-7,14).

Another important advantage of these chemiluminescent probe-methods is the optimalization of radical-scavenger mixtures. In our laboratories this optimalization focused new light upon the role of toxic cellular oxidations and their theraputic inhibition. This is of particular interest in the study of rheumatism, cancer, inflammation, DNA damage and cerebral ischemia (4) and especially, gerontology, where the "free radical theory of aging" dominates (3).

Cellular Defense Systems and Active Oxygens

Aerobic organisms generate active oxygens as biproducts of metabolism. These chemically reactive biproducts are rendered harmless by elaborate defense mechanisms. Figure 1 depicts five lines of defense in man which progressively defend the cell against damage from superoxide and its daughter active-oxygens.

Each line of defense detoxifys only a part of the total, steady-state concentration of active oxygens. Furthermore, many lines of defense must be regenerated continually following their steady-state reactions with active oxygens. This regeneration occurs by three possible methods:
1) Extracellular antioxidant nutrients must penetrate the different mitochondrial membranes and compartments in order to regenerate a membrane-bound, line-of-defense molecule. These nutrients, i.e. mercaptoamino acids, must have higher redox potentials and/or significantly higher concentrations locally in a given mitochondrial compartment in order to reduce a given, membrane-bound, line-of-defense molecule back to its active state.
2) Extracellular antioxidants are linked to other antioxidants in a redox chain with favorable equilibriums (Fig.2). This redox chain has reductive mediators which induce regeneration of primary line-of-defense molecules without the necessity of membrane penetration by nutrients.

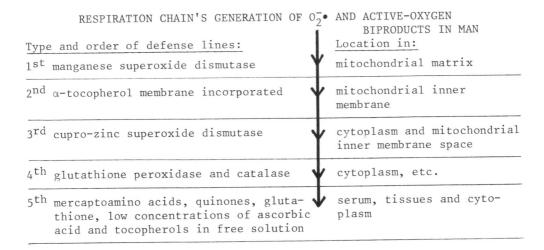

RESPIRATION CHAIN'S GENERATION OF $O_2^-\bullet$ AND ACTIVE-OXYGEN BIPRODUCTS IN MAN

Type and order of defense lines:	Location in:
1st manganese superoxide dismutase	mitochondrial matrix
2nd α-tocopherol membrane incorporated	mitochondrial inner membrane
3rd cupro-zinc superoxide dismutase	cytoplasm and mitochondrial inner membrane space
4th glutathione peroxidase and catalase	cytoplasm, etc.
5th mercaptoamino acids, quinones, glutathione, low concentrations of ascorbic acid and tocopherols in free solution	serum, tissues and cytoplasm

FIG. 1. Cellular lines of defense in man which inactivate active oxygens generated *in vivo*.

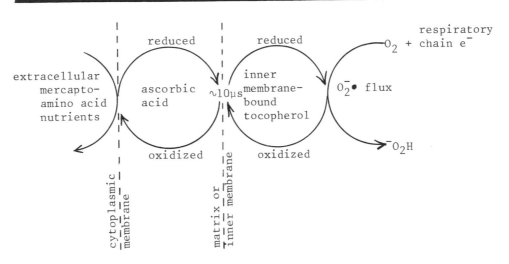

FIG. 2. A proposed redox chain for antioxidants and membrane-bound lines of defense in highly compartmentalized mitochondria. *In vitro* reduction of α-tocopherol by ascorbic acid in excess concentration takes ∿10µs. The half-life of an α-tocopherol radical intermediate is rather long, namely ∿3 ms. A word of caution: in low concentrations, ascorbic acid acts as a antioxidant mediator while in very high concentrations, it acts as a pro-oxidant and the redox chain is presumably thrown out of function.

3) A third method which artificially induces regeneration is by extra-cellular compounds which alter membrane integrities and permeabilities. One example is dimethyl sulfoxide (DMSO) which is known to scavenge •OH radicals in non-cellular *in vitro* experiments. But according to our experiments, its dominating role with mitochondria is to increase membrane permeability which in turn increases the flow of extramitochondrial anti-oxidants and nutrients. A second example is high concentrations of as-

corbic acid which are prooxidative and lysate and/or disrupt membrane integrities (7,8). This is in contrast to low concentrations which do not
lead to membrane dysfunction.

These descriptions of regeneration are admittedly sketchy. Future research is needed which coordinates different experimental skills in chemistry and medicine.

Cellular Defense Systems Among Different Species

Table 1 compares the different lines of defense against active oxygens
in different species. Notice that these lines of defense become more refined and elaborate as the evolutionary scale is advanced.

TABLE 1. Species-specific distributions of superoxide dismutases(SOD)and
other important active-oxygen inhibiting enzymes and substrates

Location	E.Coli	Rat	Chicken	Baboon	Human
Mitochondrial Matrix		~90% Mn-SOD[13]	~60% Mn-SOD[15]	some Mn-SOD[9]	Mn-SOD~20X more than in rat[12,15]
Mitochondrial Inner Membrane		Vit.E[11]			Vit. E[11]
Mitochondrial Inner Membrane Space		~86%[13] CuZnSOD	~99%CuZn[10] ~29%Mn-SOD[15]	CuZn-SOD[9]	
Cytoplasm	Fe-SOD[9]	CuZn-SOD[1] Xanthine-oxidase[2]		mostly Mn-SOD[9]	less CuZn-SOD than in rat[9]
Outer Membrane of the cell		~61% mono-amine oxidase[13]			

One prominent example which illustrates these differences is in the
case of manganese superoxide dismutase (Mn-SOD). Mn-SOD concentration in
the mitochondrial matrix is approximately 20 times higher in man than in
rat (11,15). This means that the first and foremost line of defense, Mn-
SOD, is far more efficient in dismutating $O_2^-\bullet$ and in inhibiting its
ter active-oxygens in man. This fact may partially account for man's
longer lifespan and reduced rate of aging relative to other mammals.

Man's lines of defense against active oxygens are highly compartmentalized with membrane-bound,active-oxygen detoxifiers often in close molecular proximity to active-oxygen sources of production (8). Our carni-
tinylmaleate-isoluminol probe (CML) has detected $O_2^-\bullet$ and $\bullet OH$ fluxes from
the inner membrane of intact mitochondria during state 3 respiration(5).
Our site-specific, enzyme-specific SDLG probe detected free radicals and
β-glucuronidase activity in lysosomes of intact glial cells (7). Such
probes might be used in the study of suspected free-radical activators in
endocrine cells.

Suspected Free-Radical Activators in Pancreatic β-Cells

Alloxan and streptozotocin induce diabetes and destruction of pancreatic β-Cells in experimental animals. The exact toxic mechanism is unknown. One possible hypothesis might be based upon the premise that these compounds induce high rates of oxidative metabolism, hormone production, and consequently, high fluxes of active oxygens. This is certainly the case in mild, sub-diabetic rats. Furthermore, β-cells may not have the elaborate lines-of-defense to cope with high active-oxygen flux as is the case in liver cells. Consequently, a metabolism-induced self-destructive mechanism is a possibility.

CONCLUSIONS

Inhibitors and scavengers are important in homeostatically maintaining figure one's five lines of defense in redox states that are predominately reductive and not oxidative. These highly compartmentalized redox systems primed with extracellular, reductive nutrients or redox mediators succumb ubiquitously to dysfunctions when they are not continually primed with extracellular, reductive nutrients *in vivo*. They are of interest in the study of endocrine cells which often exhibit high rates of metabolism and consequent high fluxes of active oxygens.

Supported by The Swedish Medical Research Council (Project No. B81-12X-00525) and The Swedish Natural Science Research Council (Project No. K-UR 2741-105).

REFERENCES

1. Baudhuin, P., Peeters-Joris, C. and Vandevoorde, A.M.(1975):Subcellular localization of superoxide dismutase in rat liver. Biochem.J., 150: 31-39.

2. Fridovich, I. and Handler, P. (1961): Detection of free radicals generated during enzymic oxidations by the initiation of sulfite oxidation. J. Biol. Chem., 236: 1836-1840.

3. Harman, D. (1969): Prolongation of life: Role of free radical reactions in aging. J. Amer. Ger. Soc., 17:721-735.

4. Lewis, D.H. and Del Maestro, R.(1980): Free radicals in medicine and biology, edited by D.H. Lewis and R. Del Maestro, Acta Phys. Scand., Uppsala.

5. Lippman, R.D. (1980): Chemiluminescent measurement of free radicals and antioxidant molecular-protection inside living rat-mitochondria. Exp. Geront., 15:339-352.

6. Lippman, R.D. and Ågren, A. (1981): Direct determination of pH and ATP/respiratory coupling internally in rat mitochondria with bio- and chemiluminescence. Bio. Biophys. Acta., in press.

7.   Lippman, R.D., Ågren, A. and Uhlén, M. (1981): A new method which investigates lysosomal sensitivity to superoxide with endocytotic, site-specific chemiluminescent probes. Mech. Ageing Dev., in press.

8.   Lippman, R.D., Ågren, A. and Uhlén, M. (1981): Application of chemi-luminescent probes in investigating lysosomal sensitivity to superoxide versus suspected radical scavengers. Mech. Ageing Dev., in press.

9.   McCord, J.M., Boyle, J.A., Day Jr., E.D. Rizzolo, L.J. and Salin, M. (1977): A manganese-containing superoxide dismutase from human liver.In: Superoxide and superoxide dismutases, edited by A.M. Michelson, J.M. Mc-Cord and I. Fridovich, pp. 129-138, Academic Press, New York.

10.   Panchenko, L.F., Brusov, O.S., Gerasimov, A.M. and Loktaeva, T.D. (1975): Intramitochondrial location and release of rat liver superoxide dismutase. FEBS Let., 55:84-87.

11.   Pryor, W.A. and Mead, J.F. (1976): The role of free radical reactions in biological systems. Free radical mechanisms of lipid damage and conse-quences for cellular membranes. In: Free radicals in biology, edited by W.A. Pryor, pp. 1-68, Academic Press, New York.

12.   Taylor, S.L., Lamden, M.P. and Tappel, A.L. (1976): Sensitive fluor-ometric method for tissue tocopherol analysis. Lipids, 11:530-538.

13.   Tyler, D.D. (1975): Polarographic assay and intracellular distribu-tion of superoxide dismutase in rat liver. Biochem. J., 147: 493-504.

14.   Uhlén, M. and Lippman, R.D. (1981): Kan åldrandet försenas? Forsk-ning och Framsteg, 1:24-27.

15.   Weisiger, R.A. and Fridovich, I. (1973): Mitochondrial superoxide dismutase. Site of synthesis and intramitochondrial localization. J.Biol. Chem., 248:4793-4796.

Luminescent Assays: Perspectives in Endocrinology and Clinical Chemistry, edited by M. Serio and M. Pazzagli, Raven Press, New York © 1982.

Chemiluminescence in the Peroxidation of Noradrenaline and Adrenaline

D. Sławinska and J. Sławinski

Institute of Physics and Chemistry, Agricultural University, 60-637 Poznań, Poland

Physiological hormones and drugs with dihydroxyphenylethylamine structures, such as dopamine, DOPA, adrenaline etc are converted by the oxidative cyclization into various indole derivatives via intermediate uncyclized o-quinones. This reaction serves as the basis of a major chemical assay for catecholamines in biological sources. A considerable amount of interest has also developed in the last decade in the probability of short-lived but physiologically important intermediates being formed in the course of catecholamines oxidation (4). Recently it has been shown that oxidation of certain catecholamines and aminochromes is accompanied by weak chemiluminescence (6-8, 10-11). This phenomenon opens up a new frontier for both analytical assays and better understanding the mechanism of catecholamines activity. We have investigated a weak chemiluminescence (CL) accompanying the direct and indirect oxidation of adrenaline and noradrenaline in a simple model system. The system is pertinent to the major biochemical feature of the transformations of catecholamines both in vitro and in vivo.

MATERIALS AND METHODS

Adrenaline, noradrenaline and horseradish peroxidase were from Koch and Light. Other reagents were of analytical grade from POCh Gliwice, Poland. Stock solutions (5 μM) of the catecholamines were prepared in 10 uM HCl and twice-distilled water to ensure stability. The intensity of CL was measured using an RCA 5596 A photomultiplier with an S-11 photocathode (350-650 nm). The standard concentrations of substrates in the reaction mixture were as follows: 1 mM catecholamine, 0,1 M peroxide, 5 mM ferricyanide or 0.2 μM peroxidase and 40 mM ammonium acetate buffer. The reproducibility of chemiluminescence peak heights was about 15-20% and each measurement was repeated four to six times. Details are given elsewhere (11). The reaction course was also followed spectrophotometrically and fluorometrically by measuring the characteristic absorption band of aminochromes at about 490 nm and fluorescence excitation and emission peaks of catecholamines at 260-275 nm and 315-330 nm, respectively.

RESULTS

The effect of substrate concentrations, the sequence of their mixing, catalysts, pH and temperature on the CL intensity and the absorbance of aminochromes has been studied in a series of preleminary experiments.

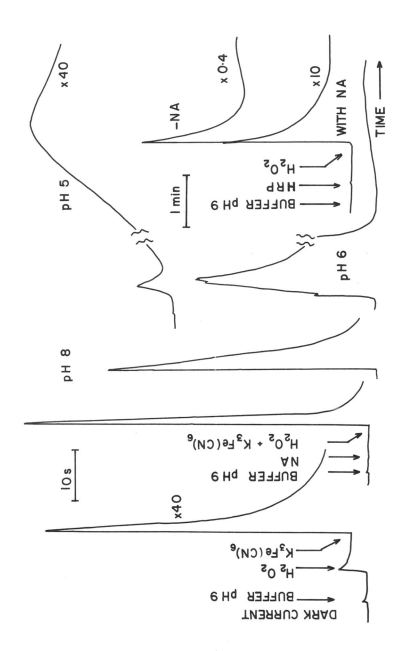

FIG. 1. Kinetics of chemiluminescence in the direct and indirect peroxidation of noradrenaline

No CL has been observed until the oxidative cyclization of catecholamines to the corresponding aminochromes occured. Catecholamines themselves effectively quenched CL generated by the system H_2O_2 + $K_3Fe(CN)_6$ + OH^- or H_2O_2 + horseradish peroxidase (HRP). This is clearly evident from the comparison of two kinetic curves I = f(t) for the indirect peroxidative system with HRP in the presence and absence of noradrenaline (Fig. 1). The same is valid for other catecholamines like adrenaline and DOPA. However, if the formation of aminochrome is very fast, then the presence of catecholamine in the reaction mixture enhances light intensity. This case is illustrated by the two first kinetic curves in Fig 1. Ferricyanide as a proper one-electron acceptor (E'_o = 0.36 V) directly and rapidly oxidizes noradrenaline to the corresponding aminochrome (pH = 7-9). The analogous reaction with adrenaline proceedes much slower and this compound always quenches CL of the both systems.

In the autoxidation reaction of catecholamines the formation of aminochromes and hydrogen peroxide as a stable product of O_2 reduction take place gradually:

$$CAH_2 + O_2 \rightarrow CAH\cdot + \bar{O}_2^. + H^+$$
$$CAH_2 + \bar{O}_2^. \rightarrow CAH\cdot + H_2O_2$$
$$2\ CAH\cdot \rightarrow CAH_2 + CA\ (quinone)$$

The formation and the subsequent utilization of H_2O_2 plays a key role. Therefore the lag phase (induction period) in the accompanying CL appears and CL intensity also increases gradually. The rate of aminochrome formation and CL intensity are enhanced by the following factors: 1/ the addition of H_2O_2, 2/ the addition of catalysts like Mn^{2+}, haemin, haemoglobin, peroxidase, 3/ the presence of an electron acceptors with a proper redox potential like ferricyanide, Fe^{3+}/Fe^{2+} which stimulate the direct oxidation, 4/ the increase of pH and 5/ the increase of temperature.

As it is seen from Fig. 1 and 2, pH strongly affects the intensity and kinetics of CL. The optimum pH region with respect to I_{max} is equal to 3.6-9.5 for noradrenaline, adrenaline as well as for adrenochrome and adrenolutin (/, 10). At lower pH values the rate of aminochrome production decreases. This make it possible to separate two CL peaks both in the time scale and light intensity (see Fig. 1 and 2). For adrenaline, such a separation occurs at higher pH values (<9.5) since the rate of aminochrome formation is lower than that for noradrenaline.

Catecholamines oxidation at pH 7 was found to involve reduction of 4 equivalents of ferricyanide (transfer of four electrons) and release of 5 equivalents of H^+ (3). The linear relationship for the concentration of aminochrome or hydrogen peroxide and CL intensity may be obtained in the case of the optimized system, containing an excess of remaining substrates:

$$I_{max} \sim -\left(\frac{\Delta A_{490}}{dt}\right)_{H_2O_2} \sim [H_2O_2]\ \text{at pH = const and}\ [aminochrome] > [H_2O_2]$$

and

$$I_{max} \sim -\left(\frac{\Delta A_{490}}{dt}\right)_{H_2O_2} \sim [aminochrome]\ \text{for}\ [H_2O_2] = const > [aminochrome]$$

and pH = const.
The observed relationships and differences between noradrenaline and adrenaline oxidation rate might be a basis for chemiluminescent assay of catecholamines determination and differentiation.

From table 1 it is evident that due to the higher activation energy the reaction rate of adrenaline is slower than that of noradrenaline. At lower pH the activation energy increases which is consistent with the release of H^+ accompanying the formation of aminochromes. Changes in temperature slightly influence the shape of kinetic curves of the noradrenaline CL, while strongly differentiate that of adrenaline. Low values of E_a suggest the radical mechanism of the chemiluminescence rate -determining step.

Results of fluorescence measurements indicate the similarity, if no identity, in the autoxidation and indirect oxidation mechanism. The data of Fig. 3 firmly prove that the rate of noradrenaline transformation (λ_{ex} 270, λ_{em} 320 nm) is greater than that of adrenaline (λ_{ex} 260, λ_{em} 315 nm). After 24 h of the peroxidation with HRP in the mild conditions (pH = 7.0, T = 290 K) there is no fluorescence from noradrenaline (λ_{ex} 270 nm), while the emission from adrenaline (λ_{ex} 270, λ_{em} 225 nm) is still of considerable intensity. Multiple fluorescing products are formed in the indirect peroxidation of both catecholamines. Those with maximum emission at 425-430 nm and 475-480 nm (λ_{ex} 340-350 nm) could not be identified. Fluorescence in the region 505-535 nm (λ_{ex} 350-400 nm) originates from the strongly fluorescing

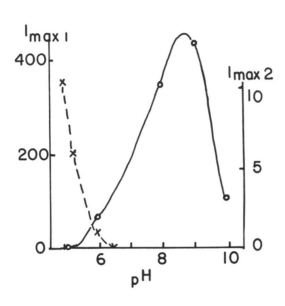

FIG. 2. The effect of pH on the maximum intensity of chemiluminescence for the noradrenaline-H_2O_2 - $K_3Fe(CN)_6$ system.

intermediate, adrenolutin (7, 10). However, this compound is unstable under the aerobic conditions and the yield of its production is low.

TABLE 1

Temperature coefficient and activation energy of noradrenaline and adrenaline chemiluminescence in the peroxidative reaction

system	pH	temperature, K	Q_{10}	E_a kJ/mole
1 mM noradrenaline	6.0	293-303	1.28	18.13
+ 10 mM H_2O_2		303-313	1.12	8.31
+ 5 mM $K_3Fe(CN)_6$	9.0	293-303	1.18	12.08
		303-313	0.98	0.75
1 mM adrenaline	9.0	293-303	1.27	18.05
+ 10 mM H_2O_2		303-313	1.05	3.63
+ 5 mM $K_3Fe(CN)_6$				

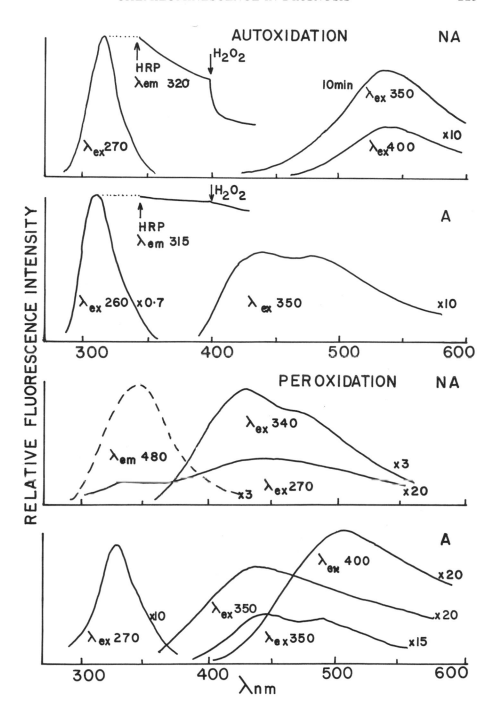

FIG. 3. Fluorescence spectra in the indirect oxidation of noradrenaline and adrenaline. Numbers at the right end of curves are sensitivity factors.

DISCUSSION

The ultimate substrates of the chemiluminescent reaction appear to be aminochrome, H_2O_2 and OH^-. The omission of any of the three substituents lead to a greatly diminished CL. The reaction is initiated by the nucle-ophilic attack of OOH^- or O_2^-, on the positively polarized carbon atom in carbonyls:

$\Delta H \simeq -265 \text{ kJ.mole}^{-1}$

The oxidative opening of the six-membered ring of indoloquinone occurs probably via a dioxetane intermediate. Electronic excited, light-emitting species are expected to be carboxylic products of this reaction. The pro-posed mechanism is supported by the following data: i/ the correlation between the increase of CL intensity and the depletion of aminochrome, caused by the addition of hydrogen peroxide, ii/ the calculation of the π-electron densities and bond orders of aminochrome molecules and, iii/ acidic character of the reaction products. In the alkaline solution the rate of the oxidative ring-opening is accelerated and the chemical yield of a strongly fluorescing adrenolutin is enhanced (7, 10, 11). This leads to the increase in CL intensity and may be used for analytical pur-poses.

Some intermediates and end-products of the aminochrome pathway are pharmacodynamically highly reactive. Cytotoxic agents like hydrogen per-oxide, superoxide anion, hydroxyls (8), singlet molecular oxygen (6, 11), o-quinones, 5,6-dihydroxyindoles (4, 7) and rheomelanins (5) are formed.

In our experiments the production of rheomelanins is confirmed by the following: i/ the absorption spectra of end-products which show a monoto-nic increase of optical density with the decrease of λ and resemble the soluble low-molecular fractions of melanins and, ii/ the ESR spectra of the end-products reaction mixture with typical "dark" and photoinduced singlet signals (g-value = 2.0048 and ΔH = 2.1 G).

Besides above mentioned analytical and toxicological aspects, the fin-dings of the work are also relevant to the possible activating and/or triggering role of electronic excited states generated in the metabolic pathways of catecholamines. It can not be excluded that excited states or photons emitted may be utilized in promoting some biochemical reactions in the nervous and hormonal functions (1, 2, 9).

The work supported by the Polish Academy of Sciences Grant no. 03.10.

REFERENCES

1. Cilento, G.: Photobiochemistry in the dark, VIII Intern. Congress Pho-tobiol. July 20-25 1980, Strassbourg, France.
2. Fischer H. A. (1979): In:Electromagnetic Bioinformation, edited by F.A. Popp and G. Becker, H. L. König, W. Peschka, pp. 175-180. Urban and Schwarzenberg, München-Wien-Baltimore.
3. Harrison, W. H., Whisler, W. W., and Hill, B. J. (1968): Biochem. 7: 3089-3094.

4. Heacock, R. A. (1971): Bull. Chem. therapetique, 4:300-304.
5. Hedegus, Z. L. and Altschule, M. D., (1970): Arch. Intern. Pharmaco-dyn. 186:39-43; 48-53.
6. Heikkila, R. E., and Cabbat, F. S., (1978): Photochem. Photobiol. 28:677-680.
7. Kruk, I., and Sławinska, D., Chemiluminescence during the oxidation of adrenaline, IV Intern. Biophys. Congress, August 7-14 1972, Moscow abstr. EIII p. 52.
8. Misra, H. P., and Fridovich, I., (1972): J. Biol. Chem. 247:3170-3175.
9. Popp, F. A., (1979): In:Electromagnetic Bioinformation, edited by F.A. Popp and G. Becker, H. L. König, W. Peschka, pp. 123-149. Urban and Schwarzenberg, München-Wien-Baltimore.
10. Sławinska, D., and Kruk, I., Luminescence of adrenaline and its deri-vatives, II Polish Luminescence Conf., Nicholas Copernicus Univ., Toruń, Poland, vol. 2:66-73; 207-215.
11. Sławinska, D., (1978): Photochem. Photobiol. 28:453-458.

Luminescent Assays: Perspectives in Endocrinology and Clinical Chemistry, edited by M. Serio and M. Pazzagli, Raven Press, New York © 1982.

Chemiluminescence Assays in the Diagnosis of Immune and Hematological Diseases

H. Fischer, M. Ernst, F.-E. Maly, *T. Kato, *H. Wokalek, **M. Heberer, †D. Maas, ††B. Peskar, §E. Th. Rietschel, and Hj. Staudinger

*Max-Planck-Institut für Immunbiologie, *Universitätshautklinik, †Medizinische Klinik, and ††Pharmakologisches Institut der Universität, Freiburg, Federal Republic of Germany; §Forschungsinstitut Borstel, Borstel, Federal Republic of Germany; **Kantonsspital, Basel, Schweiz*

In the last decades immunobiological research has mainly concentrated on the refined analysis of those cells which are involved in the specificity of the body's reactions to foreign antigens. Here lymphocytes were found to be the most important cells. More recent studies on the regulation of immune functions have brought phagocytic cells into focus. Macrophages and granulocytes, by means of receptors and their ability to produce mediators are important in the recognition of antigens and in the regulation of immune responses. Their most important function, however, is the killing, uptake and digestion of microbes, altered cells and eventually of parasites.

Pioneer studies on the initial biochemical mechanisms of killing have been performed by Babior (4), Karnovsky (5), and Klebanoff (6). They were able to demonstrate that contact with microbes or foreign material initiates a greatly enhanced oxygen consumption of phagocytes with simultaneous generation of reactive oxygen species. Univalent reduction of molecular oxygen first leads to the generation of superoxide anion (O_2^-) which subsequently disproportionates to peroxide (H_2O_2). Interactions of these activated oxygen species may yield hydroxyl radicals ($^.$OH) as well as singlet oxygen $(^1\Delta O_2)$. These oxygen species are essential for granulocyte and macrophage-mediated killing of invaders.

For monitoring oxygen activation various methods have been elaborated (4). Among them chemiluminescence (CL) measurements appear to be most simple and rapid. The emittence of photons during phagocytosis was first described by Allen et al. (1). It is based on the relaxation of electronically excited oxygen derivatives which are formed when organic material, e.g. from cell walls of bacteria is attacked by reduced oxygen. The intensity of the emitted photons is generally low; it can, however, be amplified by several orders of magnitude, when luminogenic substrates like luminol (2) (5-amino-2,3-dihydro-1,4-phtalazinedione) or lucigenin (3) (10,10' dimethyl-9,9'-biacridinium dinitrate) are present. Luminol or lucigenin therefore allow the measurement of CL with relatively few cells and cells in complex physiological fluids like whole blood (13,14).

In the following sections we will give a number of relevant examples of how CL measurements may be used in cell research and clinical diagnosis.

CALMODULIN AND MACROPHAGE CHEMILUMINESCENCE

Macrophage CL measurements have successfully been used in several laboratories for the analysis of activation followed by stimulation with phagocytic and non-phagocytic stimuli (19,20). Furthermore studies on cell interactions with lymphocytes (23,24), with tumor target cells (11) and with parasites (12) have been reported. Here I would like to present some experiments of a more general topic.

In view of the increasing evidence that calmodulin, an ubiquitous Ca^{2+} binding protein, mediates the effects of calcium in many cellular reactions (7), its impact on zymosan-induced CL was studied using bone marrow-derived mouse macrophages. As depicted in Figure 1; externally added calmodulin (8 µM) does not change subsequent zymosan-induced CL and prostaglandin synthesis.

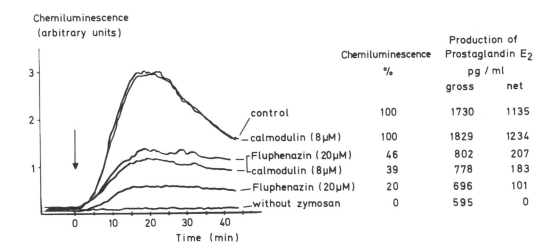

Fig. 1: Effect of calmodulin and its specific inhibitor fluphenazin on zymosan induced chemiluminescence and prostaglandin formation of bone marrow derived mouse macrophages.

2.5×10^5 macrophages were incubated in 0.5 ml of Eagle's medium buffered with HEPES at pH 7.4 (EHM medium) containing 0.04 mg/ml luminol. Calmodulin or fluphenazin were added 5 min before CL induction (arrow) by zymosan (final concentration 1 mg/ml). 40 minutes following zymosan addition supernatants were taken and stored at -20^{0}C until determination of prostaglandin E_2 by radio immuno assay.

This is in contrast to recent findings of Cheung and collaborators (22) who reported, that in platelets calmodulin induces prostaglandin and thromboxane synthesis, probably due to the prior activation of a membrane-bound Ca^{2+}-dependent phospholipase A_2. Thus, in macrophages, calmodulin does not directly induce stimulation. If the intracellular calmodulin is blocked with fluphenazin, CL and prostaglandin synthesis are strongly inhibited by rather low concentrations of the inhibitor. This inhibition, however, can be partly overcome by calmodulin (Fig. 1) indicating that in macrophages CL and prostaglandin formation are both calmodulin dependent.

Fluphenazin is a neuroleptic phenothiazine derivative. When applied locally and in higher concentrations it acts as a local anaesthetic. The question may be asked: Does a classical local anaesthetic like lidocaine also antagonize calmodulin and consequently depress zymosan-induced CL and prostaglandin synthesis in mouse macrophages ?

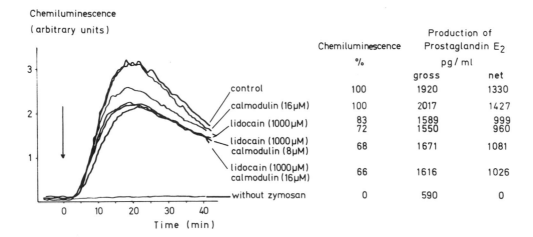

Fig. 2: Effect of calmodulin and lidocaine on zymosan induced chemiluminescence and prostaglandin formation of bone marrow derived mouse macrophages.

2.5×10^5 macrophages were incubated in 0.5 ml of EHM containing 0.04 mg/ml luminol. Calmodulin or lidocaine were added 5 min before CL induction (arrow) by zymosan (final concentration 1 mg/ml). Prostaglandins were determined as described in fig. 1.

As is shown in figure 2 this does not seem to be the case: only in very high concentrations a slight inhibitory effect on CL and prostaglandin synthesis was observed. We conclude from these experiments that lidocaine does not affect intracellular calmodulin and phospholipase A_2 in macrophages, unless very high concentrations are applied.

GRANULOCYTE CHEMILUMINESCENCE

CL measurements of isolated granulocytes have found wide applications for the detection and analysis of metabolic defects like those in chronic granulomatous disease, in myeloperoxidase deficiency, in drug induced enzyme poisoning, malnutrition and biochemical immaturity of prematurely born children (see 16).

A perhaps even wider application may be envisaged, when granulocytes (also monocytes, basophils or eosinophils) are used to recognize the presence of serum components like complement, specific antibodies and immune complexes. Doll, Merlin and Salvaggio (9) have reported, that granulocytes preexposed to either experimentally aggregated immunoglobulin or to sera from systemic Lupus erythmatodes (SLE) patients containing immune complexes, exhibit a diminished rate of CL, when subsequently challenged with opsonized zymosan. The authors claim that this inhibition might be used to develop a simple and quantitative assay for the detection of immune complexes in sera from patients.

We have chosen a different approach, namely to monitor continuously granulocyte CL following the addition of normal serum, serum plus

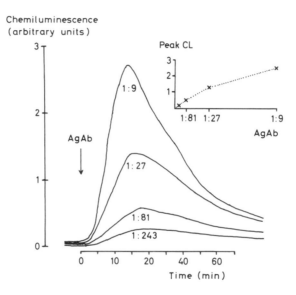

Fig. 3 Dose-dependence of antigen-antibody-complex-induced chemilumines-cence of PMN's.

Chemiluminescence of 4×10^5 PMN's suspended in 500 ul EHM containing 20 µl of fresh normal serum (as complement source) and 20 ug luminol was elicited with different dilutions of preformed antigen-antibody-complex consisting of 1 part tetanus-toxoid and 10 parts of human anti-tetanus antibody.
Insert shows nearly linear relationship between concentration of complex and peak chemiluminescence.

defined immune complexes and patient's serum. In principle all determina-tions were performed in a similar way: granulocyts from heparinized blood were isolated at $4°C$ employing a modified Böyum technique (6) and resuspended in Eagle's medium buffered with 50 mM HEPES to pH 7.4. Aliquots containing 1×10^5 cells were pipetted into the cuvettes of a Berthold Biolumat apparatus and thermostasized at $37°C$ for 10 min. Luminol was added (final concentration 0.04 mg/ml) and baseline recording started. After 10 min serum (50 µl) was added.

The granulocytes' response to antigen-antibody complexes seems to be almost identical to the CL elicited by addition of zymosan. There is, however, a great difference which becomes evident when the role of complement in both processes is analyzed. While zymosan CL is hardly affected by the absence of active complement, antigen-antibody-complex induced CL is greatly complement dependent (Fig. 4).

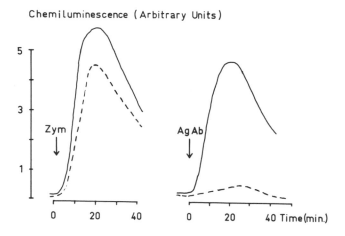

Fig. 4: Complement dependence of PMN chemiluminescence induced by zymosan or antigen-antibody-complex (AgAb).
Chemiluminescence was elicited from 1×10^5 PMN suspended in 500 ul EHM containing 50 ul of either fresh normal serum (solid line) or 50 µl of the same serum previously heated to 56°C for 30 min (dashed line) and 20 ug luminol.

We then proceeded to analyze sera from patients suffering from acute SLE and rheumatoid arthritis. The results are shown in Figure 5.

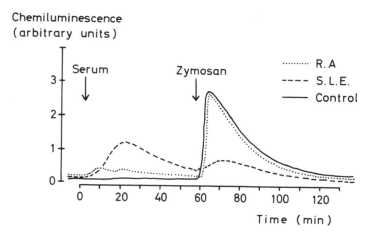

Fig. 5: To 2.5×10^5 PMN's suspended in 250 ul EHM containing 20 µg of

luminol 250 µl of serum was added to record lucigenic activity of serum. 1 hour
later zymosan was added in a final concentration of 1 mg/ml.

The dashed line was obtained with the serum of a 30 year old female
patient, suffering from systemic lupus erythematodes since 1972. At the time
of examination she had an acute exacerbation of SLE with fever, polyarthritis
and progessive cerebral and renal symptoms. Antinuclear antibodies and
antibodies to native DNA were strongly positive, the values of C4 and C3 were
very low.

The dotted curve was obtained with the serum of a male patient, aged 58
years, suffering from active classical rheumatoid arthritis with multiple subcu-
taneous nodules. Rheumatoid factor was positive with a titer of 1024 in the
Waaler-Rose test. The patient had a high sedimentation rate (143/153), moderate anaemia (Hb 10,3 g%) and hypergammaglobulinnemia (32%).

The solid curve was obtained with control serum from a healthy donor.

In Freiburg patients with SLE have been followed for a number of years. One
case seemed of special interest (Figs. 6 and 7). Fig. 6 shows the CL response of
3 serum samples taken at different time from a female patient with SLE since
1974.

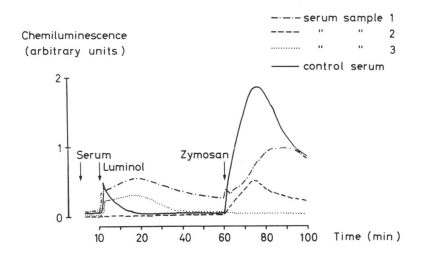

Fig. 6: Chemiluminescence elicited from PMN of a healthy donor with sera
from one patient with SLE (Ma.S.) from clinically active (samples 1 and 3, dash-
dotted and dotted lines) and inactive stages of the disease (sample 2, dashed
line). 2.5×10^5 PMN, suspended in 250 µl EHM, were incubated with 250 µl of
serum. 5 min. later luminol (20 µg) was added to record lucigenic activity of the
sera. Zymosan was added 1 hour later.

Fig. 7 gives a summary of the clinical course of her disease.

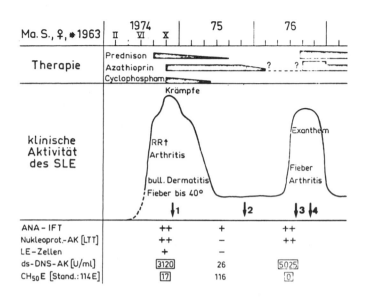

Fig. 7: Clinical course of a case of systemic lupus erythematodes.

Arrows 1-3 below the curve expressing activity of the disease correspond to serum samples 1-3 in fig. 6.

The young girl had multisystemic involvement from the beginning of the disease at the age of 11 years with fever, polyarthritis, bullous skin lesions, cerebral and renal manifestations. The activity of the disease was controlled with high doses of steroids, azathioprin and later cyclophosphamide. In 1976 the patient stopped the treatment herself which led to a new exacerbation. During active phases of the disease she had high serum levels of antibodies to native DNA and markedly reduced levels of complement.

As is evident from both figures CL responses elicited by the patient's sera themselves strikingly parallel exacerbations and remission.

In summary, these first recordings indicate that granulocytes are able to detect and possibly also to analyze the composition of preformed immune complexes in serum.

MEASUREMENTS OF CHEMILUMINESCENCE IN WHOLE BLOOD

In an attempt to make CL measurements available for routine diagnosis and for a rapid detection of a defective or abnormal defence situation we have measured zymosan-induced luminol aided CL in freshly drawn heparinized and HEPES buffered venous blood from healthy donors and from patients (13,14).

With blood from healthy donors it was found that CL curves from individuals varied considerably; this variation was, however, greatly diminished, when the curves and counts were corrected to the number of granulocytes present. This correlation at the same time proved that granulocytes are indeed the main source of zymosan-induced activated oxygen species (Fig. 8).

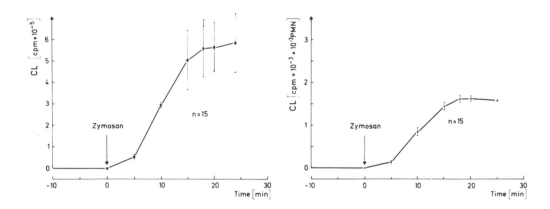

Fig. 8: Variation of zymosan-induced chemiluminescence in diluted whole blood from healthy donors.

100 μl freshly drawn whole blood were diluted by addition of 400 μl of EHM containing 0.04 mg/ml luminol. CL was induced by addition of zymosan (final concentration 1 mg/ml). Left: CL related to 100 μl whole blood. Right: CL related to the actual number of PMN's in 100 μl whole blood.

In a next step the influence of erythrocyte count variations on whole blood CL was studied. Results are shown in fig. 9.

As is evident, the presence of erythrocytes depresses the yield of measurable chemiluminescence. The variation of hematocrit in healthy donors is relatively small and does not affect CL values to an amount which deserves individual correction. Only in cases of severe anemia or polycythaemia such a correction should be made.

This standard method was used by one of us (M.H.) to analyze blood from patients of the Kantonsspital. A most unexpected finding which certainly deserves refined and detailed analysis, was the following.

Table 1: Zymosan-induced blood chemiluminescence of healthy volunteers and tumor bearing patients

Group	Cases Investigated	Chemiluminescence
	n	$cpm/10^3 PMN$ + s.d.
Control	39	15.9 $\pm$ 6.4
Malignoma	44	37.0 $\pm$ 17.3

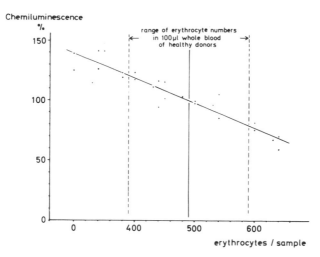

All samples contained 75μl of whole blood and were
supplemented with different numbers of erythrocytes.

Fig. 9: Influence of erythrocytes on zymosan induced chemiluminescence of diluted whole blood from 3 healthy donors.

All samples contained 75 μl of whole blood and in addition cellular blood volume corresponded to that of 100 μl whole blood. Then the samples were supplemented with different numbers of erythrocytes (blood group O). Final volume of 0.5 ml was adjusted by dilution with EHM containing 0.04 mg/ml luminol. CL was induced by addition of zymosan (final concentration 1 mg/ml). Experimental points represent the percentage of peak chemiluminescence corresponding to the samples containing 490 millions of erythrocytes. The linear regression line has a correlation coefficient of $r^2 = 0.90$.

The comparison of photon counts calculated per 10^3 granulocytes showed in tumor-bearing patients significantly higher responses than in a control population. It should be mentioned that most of those patients suffered from gastrointestinal tumors, none of them was under therapy.

Also, 6 medical students participated in a study concerning the circadian rhythm of granulocytes function man as monitored by zymosan-induced CL in whole blood. The intensity of CL was most expressed at approximately 10 a.m. in the morning and 12 hours later at 10 p.m. These results differ significantly from those obtained in mice. The latter will be reported in this symposium (17).

To close this chapter on Cl measurements in freshly drawn whole blood we would like to exemplify another application with the case of a patient suffering from sporotrichosis: a shepherd, 45 years of age, was suffering for months from multiple granuloma, predominantly in the inguinal region. Sporotrichon schenckii was isolated from these lesions and a successful treatment with ketoconazol and potassium iodide was started. Blood samples taken at various stages of the cure were analyzed by adding the specific antigen: Sporotrichon schenckii. As shows Fig. 10. The patient's blood exhibited an increased CL response to the antigen in the acute stage of his disease. During treatment CL declined and finally reached control values. This case shows that by stimulation of whole blood with appropriate specific antigens the presence and dissappearance of specific opsonins can be monitored. This might become important for the control of chronic fungal and parasitic infections.

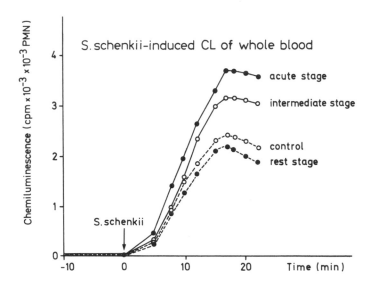

Fig. 10: S.schenckii-induced CL in whole blood of a patient with sporotrichosis and a healthy donor as control.

PLATELET-GRANULOCYTE INTERACTION IN STANDING BLOOD

To measure CL in whole blood, venous blood has to be used shortly following venipuncture. If blood is permitted to stand for one or two hours, enhanced chemiluminescence is recorded. A typical experiment with blood samples of donors is shown in Fig. 11.

In order to explain this phenomenon blood fractions were tested for zymosan-induced CL by means of separation and reconstitution experiments, which will be described in detail elsewhere (15), it was found that neither granulocytes nor platelets alone suspended in plasma undergo a change during incubation in vitro. However, if erythrocytes or factors derived thereof are present in standing heparinized blood an aggregation of platelets is seen (Fig. 12) which occurs predominantly in the neighbourhood of granulocytes (18).

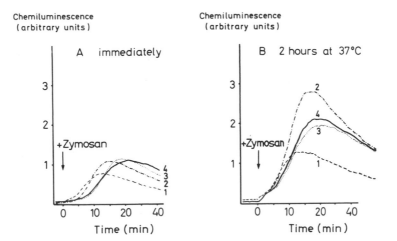

Fig. 11: Effect of incubation of blood samples on subsequent zymosan-induced chemiluminescence. Blood from 4 healthy donors was diluted 1:5 with EHM containing 0.04 mg/ml luminol and CL was induced by addition of zymosan (final concentration 1 mg/ml) either immediately after venipuncture (A) or after a 2 h incubation at 37°C (B).

a   b

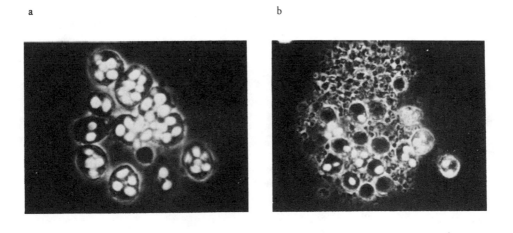

Fig. 12: a: granulocytes from freshly drawn blood after ingestion of fluorescein-conjugated zymosan
b: granulocytes with adherend aggregates of activated platelets from blood incubated for 2 hrs at 37°C after zymosan challenge.

This morphological observation demonstrates that platelets and granulocytes in standing blood are in close contact and respond to added zymosan for still unexplored reasons with enhanced CL. It is possible, however, that in standing blood in <u>vitro</u> erythrocytes release ADP which will cause platelet activation. A strong argument in favour of this explanation is given by experiments in which apyrase, an ADP-degrading enzyme, was added to blood samples. Apyrase consistently prevented platelet aggregation and also the enhancement of zymosan induced CL (cf. fig. 13).

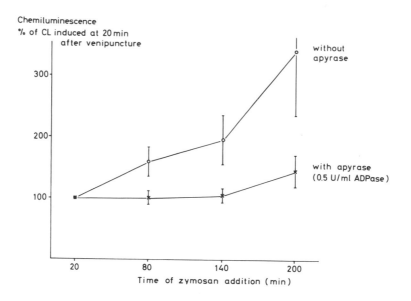

Fig. 13: Effect of apyrase on the incubation effect of blood samples on subsequent zymosan induced CL.

Blood from 4 healthy donors was diluted 1:5 with EHM containing 0.04 mg/ml luminol. The samples were incubated at 37°C either with apyrase or no supplement. CL was induced by addition of zymosan (final concentration 1 mg/ml). Peak CL of either blood source and treatment obtained following zymosan induction at time point 20 min after venipuncture was set 100%. There was an inhibitory effect of apyrase treatment on zymosan induced CL of freshly drawn whole blood of about 40% (not shown in this figure).

What we have seen in standing blood - namely platelet-granulocyte interaction leading to enhanced CL - might also occur in vivo and have clinical implications.

Acknowledgements

This work was in part supported by a grant from the Stiftung Volkswagenwerk. T. Kato is a fellow of the Alexander v. Humboldt-Stiftung. We thank Dr. D. Marmé, Institut für Biologie II, Universität Freiburg, for a generous gift of pure calmodulin.

References:

1. Allen, R.C., Stjernholm, R.L., Steele, R.H. (1972): Biochem. Biophys. Res. Comm., 47: 679-684.
2. Allen, R.C. and Loose, L.D. (1976): Biochem. Biophys. Res. Comm., 69: 245-252.
3. Allen, R.C. (1981): In: Bioluminescence and chemiluminescence. Edited by Marlene A. DeLuca and W.D. McElroy. pp. 63-73. Academic Press, New York.
4. Babior, B.M. (1978): N. Engl. J. Med., 298: 659-668, 721-725.
5. Badwey, J.A., Karnovsky,M.L. (1980): Ann. Rev. Biochem., 49: 695-726.
6. Böyum, A. (19): Scand. J. Clin. and Lab. Invest., 21, suppl. 97, 1968.
7. Cheung, W.Y. (1980): Science 207: 19-27.
8. Van Dyke, K., van Dyke, C., Peden, D., Matamoros, M. (1981): In: Bioluminescence and chemiluminescence. Edited Marlene A. DeLuca and William D. McElroy. pp. 45-53. Academic Press, New York.
9. Doll, N.J., Wilson, M.R. and Salvaggio, J.E. (1980): J. Clin. Invest., 66: 457-464.
10. Ernst, M. (1980): Behring Inst. Mitt., 65: 55-61.
11. Ernst, M., Lang, H., Fischer, H., Lohmann-Matthes, M.-L. and Staudinger, Hj. (1981): In: Bioluminescence and chemiluminescence. Edited Marlene A. DeLuca and William D. McElroy. pp. 609-616. Academic Press, New York.
12. Fischer, H. (1978): In: The Membrane Pathobiology of Tropical Diseases. pp 219-222. Edited D.F.H. Wallach. Schwabe u. Co. AG., Basel.
13. Fischer, H., Kato, T., Wokalek, H., Ernst, M., Eggert, H. and Rietschel, E.Th. (1981): In: Bioluminescence and chemiluminescence. Edited Marlene A. DeLuca and William D. McElroy. pp. 617-622. Academic Press, New York.
14. Kato, T. Wokalek, H., Schöpf, E., Eggert, H. Ernst, M., Rietschel, E.Th. and Fischer H. (1981): Klin. Wschr., 59: 203-211.
15. Kato, T., Wokalek, H., Ernst, M., Hovestadt, I. and Fischer, H. (1981): In preparation.
16. Klebanoff, S.J. and Clark, R.A. (1978): The Neutrophil, function and disorders. North-Holland Publ. Amsterdam/New York.
17. Knyszynski, A. and Fischer, H. (1981): Symposium 5.-7.7. Florence.
18. Warlow, Chr., Corina, A., Ogston, D. and Douglas, A.S. (1974): Thrombos. Diathes. Haemon., 31: 133-141.
19. Weidemann, M.J., Peskar, B.A., Wrogemann, K., Rietschel, E.T., Staudinger, Hj. and Fischer, H. (1978): FEBS Letters, 89: 136.140.
20. Weidemann, M.J., Smith, R., Heaney, T. and Alaudeen, S. (1980): Behring Inst. Mitt., 65: 42-54.
21. Wokalek, H., Kato, T. and Schöpf, E. (1980): unpublished observations.
22. Wong, P.Y.K. and Cheung, W.Y. (1979): Biochem. and Biophys. Res. Comm., 90: 473-480.
23. Wrogemann, K., Weidemann, M.J., Peskar, B.A., Staudinger, Hj. Rietschel, E.T. and Fischer, H. (1978): Eur. J. Immunol., 8: 749-752.
24. Wrogemann, K., Weidemann, M.J., Ketelsen, U.-P., Wekerle, H. and Fischer, H. (1980): Eur. J. Immunol., 10 36-40.

*Luminescent Assays: Perspectives in
Endocrinology and Clinical Chemistry*, edited by
M. Serio and M. Pazzagli, Raven Press,
New York © 1982.

Circadian Rhythm of Phagocytic Cells in Blood, Spleen, and Peritoneal Cavity of Mice as Measured by Zymosan-Induced Chemiluminescence

Ahuva Knyszynski and *Herbert Fischer

*Department of Membrane Research, The Weizmann Institute of Science, Rehovot 76100, Israel;
*Max-Planck-Institut fuer Immounobiologie, 78 Freiberg,
Federal Republic of Germany*

When phagocytic cells, such as granulocytes or macrophages are activated by phagocytosis of bacteria or zymosan particles they emit light (chemiluminescence) which can be easily measured (3,12,18,22). This chemiluminescence is considered indicative for the generation of reactive species of oxygen which emit light in the presence of polyunsaturated fatty acids, polysaccharides or easily oxidizable substances like luminol (2).

We have used the luminol-aided zymosan-induced chemiluminescence to explore the circadian rhythm in the phagocytic activity of mouse whole blood, spleen and peritoneal cells.

Circadian rhythms are documented for several biological variables including among others antibody formation to sheep red blood cells (7) rejection of skin (8) and kidney (17) allografts, resistence to endotoxins (10) and susceptibility to chemical carcinogens (9). Circadian fluctuations were also demonstrated in leukocytes, T and B cells, and natural killer cells (1,6,16), in plasma proteins such as γ globulins (19), in the complement system (14) and, recently, in the phagocytic index of reticuloendothelial system (20).

We here report circadian variations in the phagocytic activity of mouse blood, spleen and peritoneal cells.

C57Bl mice were kept in a room with light on from 7.00-19.00, alternating with darkness from 19.00-7.00 or in 2 rooms with light on from 7.00-19.00 followed by darkness in room (a) and darkness from 8.00-20.00 followed by light in room (b). At different times during the day blood was withdrawn first, then the mouse was sacrificed, spleen and peritoneal cell suspensions prepared and luminol-aided zymosan-induced chemiluminescence measured. In the beginning, our chemiluminescence measurements were performed using a Tricarb scintillation counter (Packard model 3002) in the coincidence off mode of operation and being thermostated at 37°C. At a later stage, chemiluminescence measurements were done in a Biolumat (Model LB 9505, Berthold Co., Wildbad) which allows the simultaneous and continuous measurements of 6 samples. 10^6 (if not stated otherwise) spleen or peritoneal cells or 100μl whole blood, suspended in Dulbecco's modified Eagle's medium (EM-H), were preincubated for 1h at 37ºC in either Tricarb scintillation counter or in the Biolumat counting chamber. The cell samples were then mixed with luminol and background chemiluminescence was recorded. Ten minutes later zymosan was added and chemiluminescence was continuously recorded. Count rates were calculated, and corrected by substraction of background counts.

RESULTS AND DISCUSSION

In Fig. 1 are presented results of pilot experiments in which the zymosan-induced chemiluminescence of peritoneal (a) and spleen (b) cells, prepared at different periods during 24 h , was followed. The lowest values of chemiluminescence, and therefore of phagocytic activity for both peritoneal and spleen cells were seen in cell suspensions prepared at 22.00 (3 hours after the onset of darkness). The chemiluminescence values were much higher when the cell suspensions were prepared at 4.00, 8.00 or 10.00 in the morning.

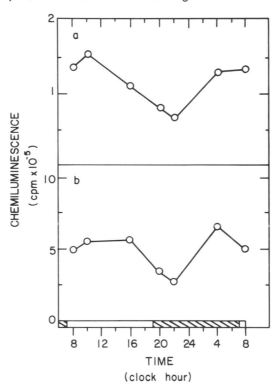

FIG. 1 Zymosan-induced chemiluminescence of peritoneal (a) and spleen (b) cells prepared at different times during a 24 hour period. 10^6 peritoneal or 10^7 spleen cells in 2.4 ml EM-H were mixed with 50μl luminol (2mg/ml) and with 25μl zymosan (50mg/ml). Chemiluminescence measurements were performed in a Packard scintillation counter. Each point on the curve represents the net rate of chemiluminescence (expressed in counts per minute) emitted by the cells 1/2 an hour after zymosan addition.

These observations suggested existance of circadian rhythm in the phagocytic activity of mouse peritoneal and spleen cells. To verify whether the results presented in Fig.1 are significant, more experiments were carried out. In these experiments cell suspensions were prepared twice a day, at the lowest period of activity i.e.at 22.00 and at 10.00, when the activity of the peritoneal and spleen cell suspensions was shown to be high. In addition to peritoneal and spleen cell suspensions, zymosan induced chemiluminescence was also measured in whole blood samples. The chemiluminescence values of all the three cell suspensions were higher when the cells were prepared at 10.00 as compared to those prepared at 22.00, the integrated counts being 82.33×10^5 and 52.76×10^5 ($p > 0.05$) for peritoneal cells, 83.3×10^5 and 32.2×10^5 ($p < 0.0001$) for spleen cells and 12.33×10^5 and 3.99×10^5 ($p < 0.001$) for blood cells (Fig.2).

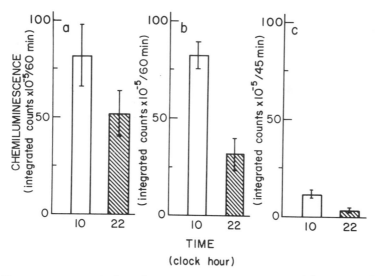

FIG.2 Zymosan induced chemiluminescence of peritoneal (a), spleen (b) and blood (c) cells prepared at 10.00 and 22.00. 10^6 peritoneal or spleen cells in 500 µl EM-H or 100 µl blood in 400 µl EM-H were mixed with 10µl luminol (2mg/ml) and with 10µl zymosan (50mg/ml). Chemiluminescence measurements were performed in the Biolumat. Results are expressed as integrated net counts per interval of 60 minutes for peritoneal and spleen cells and per interval of 45 minutes for blood samples. Mean ± S.E.M. of 16 mice for peritoneal cells, of 11 mice for spleen cells and of 12 mice for blood samples are presented. Empty columns-cell suspensions prepared at 10.00; dashed columns-cell suspensions prepared at 22.00.

In contrast to the differences in the intensity of the zymosan-induced chemiluminescence, the shapes of the curves of each cell preparation were similar, irrespective of the time period of the day the cells were prepared.

Circadian variations were also found in the leukocyte and granulocyte counts of the blood samples tested for chemiluminescence. The cell counts (leukocytes and granulocytes) of blood samples withdrawn at 10.00 were about 3 times higher as compared to the cell counts of blood samples withdrawn at 22.00 (Table 1).

TABLE 1

Blood leukocyte and granulocyte counts
at 10.00 and 22.00

Time (clock hour)	Leukocytes (x 10^4)	Granulocytes (x 10^4)
10.00	97.1 ± 9.4	18.02 ± 3.81
22.00	34.7 ± 4.0	5.15 ± 0.82
p	<0.0001	<0.001

Mean (± S.E.M.) counts per 100 µl blood for 12 mice (12 experimtns) and p values are presented.

Similar circadian variations in mice and rat blood leukocyte, eosinophil and lymphocyte counts were reported previously (1,6,11,15,16). Such significant circadian variations in the number of nucleated cells were not observed in spleen and peritoneal cell suspensions. It appears therefore that the higher chemiluminescence emitted by blood samples withdrawn from the mouse at 10.00 as compared to this seen in blood withdrawn at 22.00 is due to the differences in the number of granulocytes. Once the results are expressed as specific activity i.e. chemiluminescence counts per number of granulocytes present in the blood samples measured, the differences between morning and evening disappear. This is, however, not the case in human beings. Heberer et al. (in preparation) using the whole blood method(12), found in healthy volunteers that zymosan-induced chemiluminescence follows a highly significant circadian rhythm which is also apparent when expressed per number of granulocytes (specific activity).

Recently Szabo et al. (20) reported studies on the circadian rhythm in murine reticuloendothelial system functions. Using the carbon clearance method they observed high phagocytic activity from 8.00-22.00 followed by low activity between 2.00-6.00. Our results partially confirm the findings of Szabo et al. in so far as phagocytic activity observed by us being also high during the light phase. In contrast to their findings, in our experiments, low phagocytic activity was already apparent at the beginning of the dark phase, at 20.00 and 22.00. These partial differences between our and their results might be due to differences in techniques as well as to differences in strains of mice used.

The factors responsible for the circadian variations in the phagocytic activity described above are not known. Attention should be given to hormones and other systemic factors(4,5,13) which are secreted episodically over a relatively short period of the day. Circadian rhythm in serum corticoid levels in mice and rats are well documented (1,16,21). Possible interaction of such hormonal rhythm with phagocytic cells can occur.

Comparison of the kinetics of zymosan-induced chemiluminescence curves of spleen, blood and peritoneal cells, prepared during the same period of the day, revealed some similarity between the curves of blood and spleen cell suspensions (Fig.3). This is most probably due to granulocytes present in the spleen preparation which might be, at least partially, responsible for the fast onset of chemiluminescence seen shortly after zymosan addition. The chemiluminescence emitted by spleen cells was, however, stronger and lasted for a longer time, apparently due to macrophages present in the suspensions.

The kinetics of chemiluminescence emission of peritoneal cells differed from that of spleen and blood cells being slower at the onset, lasting for a longer time and declining slowly (Fig.3).

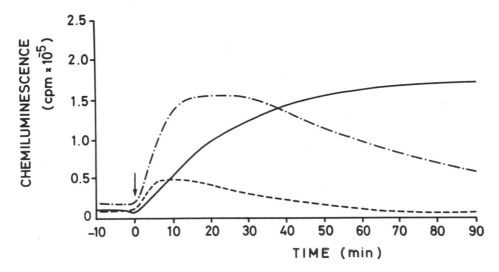

FIG. 3   The kinetics of zymosan-induced chemiluminescence of peritoneal, spleen and whole blood cells. Cell suspensions were prepared at 10.00 and the chemiluminescence emission by the cell preparations was followed in the Biolumat. Number of cells and concentrations of luminol and zymosan were the same as described in legend to Fig. 2 . —— peritoneal cells; -.-.- spleen cells; ----blood cells.

In conclusion it can be stated that chemiluminescence measurements, which can be easily performed and which monitor the pattern of the metabolic activation of a given cell type, can be applied for the demonstration and analysis of circadian rhythm.

REFERENCES

1.   Abo, T., Kawate, T., Hinuma, S., Itoh, K., Abo, W, Sato, J. and Kumagai, K. (1980): The circadian periodicities of lymphocyte subpopulations and the role of corticosteroid in human beings and mice. In: Recent Advances in the Chronobiology of Allergy and Immunology, vol. 28, edited by M.H. Smolensky, A. Reinberg and J.P.McGovern, p. 301-316, Pergamon Press.

2. Allen, R.C. and Loose, L.D. (1976): Phagocytic activation of a luminol-dependent chemiluminescence in rabbit alveolar and peritoneal macrophages. Biochem.Biophys.Res.Commun., 69: 245-252.

3. Allen, R.C., Stjernholm, R.L. and Steele, R.H. (1972): Evidence for the generation of an electronic excitation state(s) in human polymorphonuclear leukocytes and its participation in bactericidal activity. Biochem.Biophys.Res.Commun., 47: 679-684.

4. Barnes, P., Fitzgerald, G, Brown, M. and Dollery, C. (1980): Nocturnal asthma and changes in circulating epinephrine, histamine, and cortisol. N.Engl.J.Med., 303: 263-267.

5. Eckebrecht, D. and von Mayersbach, H. (1980): Circadian variations of histamine release from lungs of sensitized guinea pigs due to antigen contact. In: Recent Advances in the Chronobiology of Allergy and Immunology, Vol. 28, edited by M.H. Smolensky, A. Reinberg and J.P.McGovern, p. 317-322, Pergamon Press.

6. Fernandes, G., Halberg, F. and Good, R.A. (1980): Circadian rhythm in T,B and natural killer cells. In: Recent Advances in the Chronobiology of Allergy and Immunology, Vol. 28, edited by M.H. Smolensky, A. Reinberg and J.P. McGovern, p. 289-299, Pergamon Press.

7. Fernandes, G., Yunis, E.J., Nelson, W. and Halberg, F. (1974): Differences in immune response of mice to sheep red blood cells as a function of circadian phases. In: Chronobiology, edited by L.E.Scheving, F. Halberg and J.E. Pauly, p. 329-338, Igaku Shoin Ltd., Tokyo.

8. Halberg, J., Halberg, E., Runge, W., Wicks, J., Cadotte, L., Yunis,E., Katinas, G., Stutman, O. and Halberg, F. (1974): Transplant Chronobiology. In: Chronobiology, edited by L.E. Scheving, F. Halberg and J.E. Pauly, p. 320-328, Igaku Shoin Ltd., Tokyo.

9. Halberg, F., Haus, E. and Scheving, L.E. (1978): Sampling of biologic rhythms, chronocytokinetics and experimental oncology. In: Biomathematics and Cell Kinetics, edited by A.J.Valleron and P.D.M. Macdonald, p. 175-190, Elsevier North-Holland Biomedical Press, Amsterdam.

10. Halberg, F., Johnson, E.A., Brown, B.W. and Bittner, J.J. (1960): Susceptibility rhythm to E.coli endotoxin and bioassay. Proc.Soc.Exp. Biol.Med.,103: 142-144.

11. Halberg, F. and Visscher, M.B. (1950): Regular diurnal physiological variation in eosinophil levels in five stocks of mice. Proc.Soc.Exp.Biol. Med., 75: 846-847.

12. Kato, T., Wokalek, H., Schoepf, E., Eggert, E., Ernst, M., Rietschel, E.Th. and Fischer, H. (1981): Measurement of chemiluminescence in freshly drawn human blood. 1. Role of granulocytes, platelets, and plasma factors in zymosan-induced chemiluminescence. Klin.Wochenschr., 59: 203-211.

13. Krieger, D.T. (1979): Rhythms in CRF, ACTH and Corticosteroids. In: Comprehensive endocrinology (endocrine rhythms), edited by L. Martini, p. 123, Raven Press, New York.

14. Pallansch, M., Kim, Y., Tarquini, B., Cagnoni, M., and Halberg, F. (1980): Circadian rhythms in the human complement system. In: Recent Advances in the Chronobiology of Allergy and Immunology, Vol. 28: edited by M.H. Smolensky, A. Reinberg and J.P.McGovern, p.341-352, Pergamon Press.

15. Pownall, R., Kabler, P.A. and Knapp, M.S. (1979): The time of day of antigen encounter influences the magnitude of the immune response. Clin.Exp.Immunol., 36: 347-354.

16. Pownall, R., Knapp, M.S., Kowanko, I.C., Byme, D., Stockdale, H. and Minors, D.S. (1980): Phase relationships of corticosteroids, leukocytes and cellular immunity in vivo. In: Recent Advances in the Chronobiology of Allergy and Immunology, Vol.28: edited by M.H. Smolensky, A. Reinberg and J.P.McGovern, p. 333-339, Pergamon Press.

17. Ratte, J., Halberg, F., Kuehl, J.F.W. and Najarian, J.S., (1973): Circadian variation in the rejection of rat kidney allografts. Surgery, 73: 102-108.

18. Rozen, H. and Klebanoff, S.J., (1976): Chemiluminescence and super-oxide production by myeloperoxidase-deficient leukocytes. J.Clin.Invest., 58: 50-60.

19. Scheving, L.E., Pauly, J.E. and Tsai, T., (1968): Circadian fluctuation in plasma proteins of the rat. Am.J.Physiol., 215: 1096-1101.

20. Szabo, I., Kovats, T.G. and Halberg, F. (1978): Circadian rhythm in murine reticuloendothelial function. Chronobiologia, 5: 137-143.

21. Ungar, F. and Halberg, F. (1962): Circadian rhythm in the in vitro response of mouse adrenal to adrenocorticotropic hormone. Science, 137: 1058-1060.

22. Weidemann, M.J., Peskar, B.A., Wrogemann, K., Rietschel, E.Th., Staudinger, H.J. and Fischer, H. (1978): Prostaglandin and thromboxane synthesis in a pure macrophage population and the inhibition by E-type prostaglandins of chemiluminescence. FEBS Letters, 89: 136-140.

Luminescent Assays: Perspectives in Endocrinology and Clinical Chemistry, edited by M. Serio and M. Pazzagli, Raven Press, New York © 1982.

Functional Differentiation of Peritoneal Exudate Macrophages and Polymorphonuclear Leukocytes: An Approach Based on Chemilumigenic Probing of Phagocytic Oxygenation Response to Various Stimuli

David G. Burleson and Robert C. Allen

Department of Clinical Investigation and U.S. Army Institute of Surgical Research, Brooke Army Medical Center, Fort Sam Houston, Texas 78234

The activation of metabolism or respiratory burst that follows stimulation of phagocytic cells is characterized by increases in O_2 consumption (non-mitochondrial) and in glucose utilization via the dehydrogenases of the hexose monophosphate shunt (4). These activities are necessary for generating the oxidants capable of effecting microbicidal and cytotoxic action (1). In the present study, the oxygenation activities of two different inflammatory exudate phagocytes, macrophages (MP) and polymorphonuclear leukocytes (PMNL), were investigated by chemilumigenic probing. A chemilumigenic probe (CLP) is defined as a substrate whose oxygenation is associated with a high yield of luminescence (3). By introduction of luminol as a bystander substrate or CLP, the oxygenation activity associated with stimulation of phagocyte metabolism can be measured as chemiluminescence (CL) (2). The CLP approach to the study of oxygenation activity is ultrasensitive and nondestructive, and as such, allows continuous assessment of activity from very small numbers of phagocytes.

METHODS

Inflammation was elicited in guinea pigs by intraperitoneal injection of sodium caseinate; after 7 days, the peritoneal exudate cells were harvested by lavage, washed, placed on an eight step discontinuous gradient

---

of Percoll[R] (Pharmacia), and centrifuged at 1600 x g for 20 min. The MP were collected in the lighter fractions (d = 1.06 to 1.07), whereas the PMNL were obtained from the heaviest fraction (d = 1.08 to 1.10). The cells were washed free of Percoll and counted. Differential counts were based on cellular morphology (Wright's stain) and nonspecific esterase activity. The cells (20,000) were then added to sterile, siliconized, glass vials containing 2 ml of complete barbital buffer (Ca^{++}, Mg^{++}, albumin, and glucose added) with luminol at a final concentration of 5 μM (5). Modified liquid scintillation counters were employed for single photon counting. The instruments were equipped with high sensitivity, low dark current photomultiplier tubes (EMI 9829 AM, bialkali spectral response), and were calibrated using a blue photon emitter as standard (6). All experiments were performed at 23 ± 1°C. For each sample, CL intensity (dCL/dt), expressed as photons/min, was periodically monitored at 13 min intervals; the total photon count, integral CL, was calculated from the intensity measurements by trapezoidal approximation.

Five different stimuli were employed. Phorbol myristate acetate (PMA), a carcinogen extracted from croton oil (Sigma), and Conconavalin A (Con A), an α-methyl mannoside binding lectin isolated from jackbean (Sigma), were employed as soluble stimuli. Zymosan A (Sigma), a yeast cell wall preparation opsonified with guinea pig serum as a source of complement (OpZy), and Shigella sonnei phase I opsonified (without complement) with IgG or IgM (IgG-S.s. or IgM-S.s.) purified from antisera raised against Shigella sonnei were used as phagocytosable immune-opsonified stimuli. After two background counts of the samples, each stimulant was added to cell preparation in a 20 μl volume approximately 30 seconds before the next count.

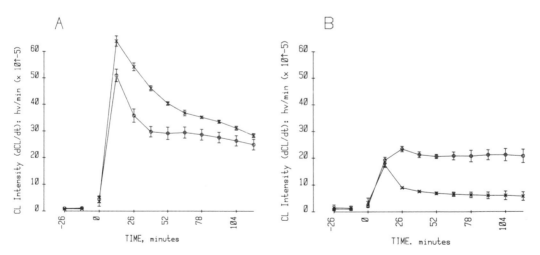

FIG. 1. Chemiluminescence intensity from the oxygenation of luminol plotted against time. MP (x——x) and PMNL (o——o) were challenged by the soluble stimuli, PMA and CON A. Each vial contained 20,000 cells in 2 ml of complete barbital buffer (pH 7.2) and 5 μl luminol. The stimuli (20 μl) were added at time 0 following 2 background counts. A) PMA (2.5 ng/ml final concentration); B) Con A (200 μg/ml final concentration). Each point represents the mean ± S.D. of four samples.

RESULTS

The luminescence responses resulting from luminol oxygenation by MP and PMNL following activation by soluble stimuli are shown in figure 1. The CL intensity is plotted against time with time zero representing the point of stimulus addition. When PMA was the stimulus, a large immediate response was elicited from both MP and PMNL (figure 1a). Addition of Con A also elicited an immediate but lesser response from both cell types (figure 1B); however, relative to the MP response, the PMNL response to Con A was greater and more sustained.

Phagocyte oxygenation activity as measured by CLP was also investigated using immune-opsonified, phagocytosable particles. The responses to serum (complement) opsonified zymosan are depicted in part A of figure 2; the responses to Shigella sonnei type I opsonified with either IgG or IgM specific for this organism are depicted in part B and C, respectively. For both MP and PMNL, the responses were delayed relative to those obtained using soluble stimuli. Both OpZy and IgG-S.s. were effective stimuli; however, OpZy was more effective as a PMNL stimulant, whereas IgG-S.s. was more effective as a MP stimulant. Using IgM-S.s., a small but detectable response was observed from PMNL, but not from MP.

For ease of comparison, the stimuli-induced responses are recapitulated in figure 3. The MP and PMNL responses are presented as part A and part B of the figure, respectively. The kinetic differences between soluble and particulate stimuli, as well as the reciprocal nature of IgG-S.s. versus OpZy, are clearly evident.

The total or integral photon count can be obtained by trapezoidal approximation of the area under each curve (2). The total photon counts from MP and PMNL for the two hour interval following addition of each of the five stimuli are presented in figure 4. The data are presented as the mean ± S.D. of 4 samples. The values obtained from unstimulated controls are presented for comparison.

DISCUSSION

Chemilumigenic probing affords an ultrasensitive technique for quantifying the oxygenation activity of as few as 10^4 phagocytes. The quantification of CL resulting from oxygenation of the CLP luminol, after challenge with selected stimuli, clearly differentiates MP from PMNL.

Heat treatment (56°C, 30 min) destroys the serum's ability to opsonify zymosan; therefore, opsonification was assumed to be effected via a phagocyte complement receptor mechanism. Shigella sonnei phase I was opsonified by purified immunoglobulin in the absence of added complement and thus stimulation was assumed to proceed via a phagocyte Fc receptor mechanism. The predominant mechanism for identification of immune opsonified particles as determined by the resulting oxygenation activity appears to be via Fc receptors for MP and complement receptors for PMNL.

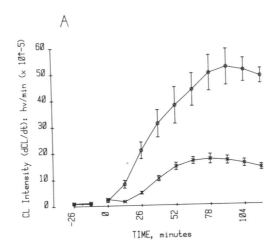

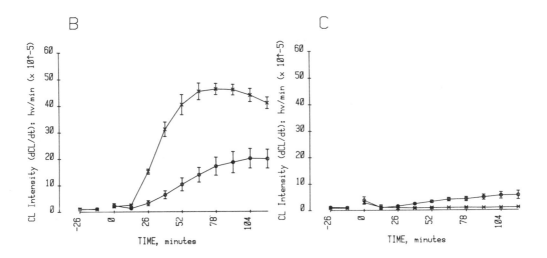

FIG. 2. Luminol-dependent CL from MP (x—x) and PMNL (o—o) challenged by particulate stimuli. Aside from the stimuli employed, conditions were the same as for FIG. 1. A) Zymosan (50 ug opsonified with 20 ul guinea pig serum. B) Shigella sonnei phase I (100 formalin-fixed bacteria per PMNL) opson- ified with immune IgG (1 ul of serum equivalent). C) Shigella sonnei phase I opsonified with immune IgM (1 ul of serum equivalent).

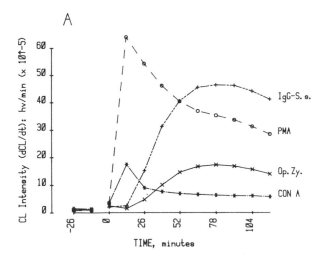

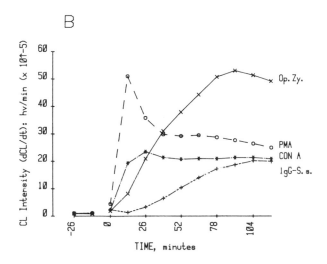

FIG. 3.   The oxygenation response of MP or PMNL to challenge
by various stimuli measured as CL intensity.   Challenge conditions are the same as FIGS. 1 and 2.   A) MP; B) PMNL.

*Luminescent Assays: Perspectives in
Endocrinology and Clinical Chemistry*, edited by
M. Serio and M. Pazzagli, Raven Press,
New York © 1982.

Determination of Hemoglobin in Serum by Iso-Luminol Chemiluminescence

T. Olsson, K. Bergström, and A. Thore

Department of Clinical Chemistry, Karolinska Institutet, Huddinge Hospital, S-141 86 Huddinge, Sweden

Acute destruction of erythrocytes results in increased plasma concentration of hemoglobin. Thus, the level of free hemoglobin in serum is of interest as an index of pathological conditions resulting in hemolysis. Mechanical treatment of blood e.g. hemodialysis may also be monitored by measuring the level of free hemoglobin. The commonly used spectrophotometric methods for determination of hemoglobin are based on the peroxidase activity of the prostethic group, protohemin, in acid solution (3, 4, 7). The coloured product is formed from a chromogenic substrate, e.g. benzidine derivatives (4, 7).

More recently chemiluminescent analysis has been used for determination of hemoglobin in clinical serum samples (5). This method was based on luminol chemiluminescence catalyzed by protohemin in alkaline solution. The sensitivity was enhanced compared to spectrophotometric methods, but samples had to be diluted so as not to overload the luminometer used to detect the emitted light.

The present study was undertaken to improve and simplify the luminol procedure. The closely related iso-luminol molecule was used as luminescent substance. The lower quantum yield of iso-luminol as compared to luminol (6) allowed the assay to be performed without extensive dilution of the serum sample.

MATERIALS AND METHODS

Reagents

Iso-luminol (4-aminophtalhydrazide) and crystalline human hemoglobin was obtained from Sigma. A standard solution of hemoglobin (70 mg/L) was prepared in deionized water. TMB (3,3',5,5'-tetramethylbenzidine) was from Aldrich. All other reagents were of analytical grade. Serum was taken from a standard pool used in routine laboratory work.

Methods

The iso-luminol assay was performed as earlier (5) with the exception that luminol was replaced by iso-luminol. The chemiluminescence was measured in an LKB 1250 Luminometer (LKB/Wallac, Turku, Finland) and the signal was registered on a 2210 Chart Recorder (LKB-Produkter AB, Bromma,

Sweden). In the final procedure a sample (10 µl) was added to 1 ml of NaOH (0.1 M), 0.2 ml of alkaline iso-luminol solution (1.2 mM) was added and the reaction was initiated by injection of 0.2 ml of Na-perborate (50 mM) by a pneumatic pipettor (Autochemist, LKB-Produkter AB, Bromma, Sweden). Each sample was also assayed with a standard addition of hemoglobin (10 µl) corresponding to 70 mg/L.

The spectrophotometric determination of hemoglobin with TMB was performed according to Standefer and Vanderjagt (7) with the modifications suggested by Geissler and Stith (2). Sample (10 µl) was added to 0.5 ml of TMB (5 mg/ml in 90% acetic acid) and the peroxidase activity initiated by addition of 0.5 ml of H_2O_2 (1%). Following 25 min incubation (25 °C) the reaction was stopped by addition of 5 ml of acetic acid (10%). The colour was measured at 375 nm. Each serum sample was also assayed with a standard addition of hemoglobin (10 µl) corresponding to 70 mg/L.

RESULTS AND DISCUSSION

Time Course of the Light Emission

The time course of the light emission from a complete reaction mixture with added serum containing hemoglobin is presented in figure 1. The time course was similar to that induced by crystalline hemoglobin in the luminol system (1). The most obvious difference was that the reaction was slower and maximum light emission reached only after 20-30 seconds. The maximum light emission was the most convenient parameter for quantitating the reaction and has been used in all subsequent experiments.

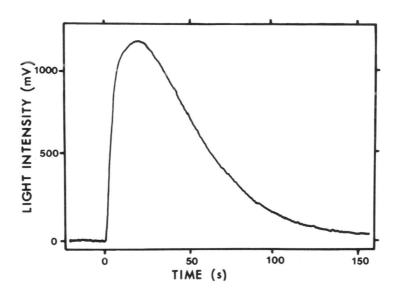

FIG. 1. The time course of the light emission induced by hemoglobin in serum using the iso-luminol system. The hemoglobin serum concentration was about 100 mg/L.

Influence of Iso-Luminol and Perborate Concentrations

The influence of iso-luminol and perborate concentrations was investigated in the next set of experiments (fig. 2). At low iso-luminol concentration there was a direct proportionality between light emission and iso-luminol concentration. At iso-luminol concentrations above 10^{-4} M the reaction approached saturation. The time course was essentially not influenced by the iso-luminol concentration. A concentration of 1.7 x 10^{-4} M iso-luminol was used in subsequent experiments.

The light emission induced by varying the concentration of perborate showed a direct proportionality over the investigated range. With increasing perborate concentration the rate of the decrease of the light emission was increased. Thus, the resulting amount of light was essentially constant independent of the perborate concentration. In subsequent expe-

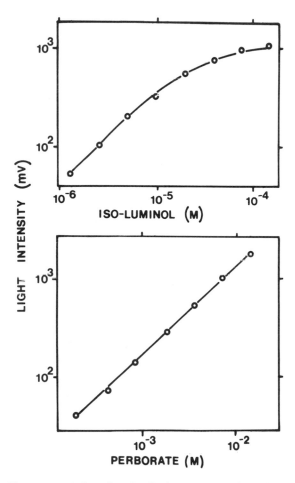

FIG. 2. The influence of iso-luminol (upper part) and perborate concentration (lower part) on the light emission in the assay of serum hemoglobin (100 mg/L). The concentrations are concentrations in the reaction mixture.

riments a perborate concentration of 7.1 mM was used resulting in con-
veniently measurable levels of light emission.

Influence of the Serum Volume

The added serum volume was varied in the next experiment (table 1).
The light emission was not increased with increasing serum volume in the
expected manner. The reason was clarified by assaying serum together
with a constant amount of added hemoglobin. Inhibition of the luminescent reaction induced by added hemoglobin was dramatically increased
with increasing serum volume. The strong inhibition caused by serum has
also been observed in the luminol system (5).
By using the added hemoglobin as an internal standard the original content of hemoglobin in the analyzed serum could be calculated. The difference in light emission between serum and serum with added hemoglobin
was used to convert the light emission from serum alone to hemoglobin
equivalents. This calculation was carried out for all serum volumes and
the calculated content of hemoglobin was found to be essentially constant irrespective of serum volume. A serum volume of 10 µl was used in
subsequent experiments.

Table 1. The influence of serum volume on determination of serum hemoglobin by iso-luminol chemiluminescence. The added standard (10 µl) contained 0.7 µg of hemoglobin.

Serum volume (µl)	Maximum light emission (mV)			Calculated hemo-globin in serum (mg/L)
	Serum (A)	Serum + Standard (B)	Standard (A-B)	
5	355	2600	2245	22.1
10	400	1650	1250	22.4
15	333	1038	705	22.0
25	302	675	373	22.7

Analysis of Hemoglobin in Serum

The analysis of different concentrations of hemoglobin in serum is presented in figure 3. For comparison hemoglobin was also measured by the
spectrophotometric TMB method. Variation of hemoglobin content was achieved by adding dilutions of a standard hemoglobin solution to a control
serum. Both methods resulted in intervals with direct proportionality
but the linear range was considerably wider using the iso-luminol method.
The control serum used contained traces of hemoglobin (5 mg/L). Concentrations of added hemoglobin was measured against this background level. Thus, under these conditions both methods had a relatively narrow
range of linearity. The actual sensitivity of the iso-luminol method as
judged from separate control experiments corresponded to 10 µg/L of serum whereas the TMB method had a limit of sensitivity of 3 mg/L.
The sensitivity and some other characteristics of the two methods are
presented in table 2. The iso-luminol method was considerably more sensitive as discussed before and also resulted in better precision.
Results from a limited number of sera indicated that the sensitivity

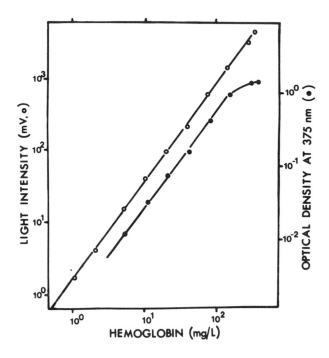

FIG. 3. Quantitation of hemoglobin in serum by the iso-luminol method
(o) and the TMB method (●). Presented hemoglobin concentrations were prepared by additions of hemoglobin to serum. Results have been corrected
for light emission or formation of colour induced by the hemoglobin present in serum before the additions.

Table 2. Some characteristics of the iso-luminol and TMB methods for determination of hemoglobin in serum.

	Iso-luminol	TMB
Dynamic range	0.01-500 mg/L	3-200 mg/L
Precision within 5-50 mg/L[1]	7.8%	10.6%
Inhibition of the chemical reaction by serum[2]	98-99.5%	20-30%
Approximate time for one assay	1 min	30 min

1) Average for determinations at 5, 20, and 50 mg/L (n=10,C.V.%)
2) Estimated range of inhibition using different sera and comparing
the light emission induced by hemoglobin standards in the absence and
presence of serum.

was sufficient for both the iso-luminol and TMB methods if tests were performed on blood which had been drawn routinely. Serum levels of hemoglobin in these blood samples were not below 5 mg/L. However, if blood was drawn with special care so as not to cause mechanical lysis of erythrocytes, levels were frequently below the limit of sensitivity of the TMB method.

The inhibitory effect of serum or serum components was found to vary slightly between different sera (table 2). This was most pronounced for the iso-luminol method. Nevertheless, individual calibrations of samples by use of an internal standard is necessary for accurate results with both methods.

The time for each assay was considerably shorter with the iso-luminol method. This allows monitoring of the lytic process which may be of importance for many applications e.g. during mechanical treatment of blood (hemodialysis).

Work is now under way to evaluate the iso-luminol method using clinical material and to compare results with conventional spectrophotometric methods.

ACKNOWLEDGEMENTS

The skillful technical assistance of Mrs. Christina Sällquist is gratefully acknowledged. This work was supported by a grant from the Swedish Board for Technical Development.

REFERERENCES

1. Ewetz, L., and Thore, A. (1976): Anal. Biochem., 71:564-570.
2. Geissler, U.C., and Stith, W.J. (1977): A Safe, Sensitive Procedure for Measuring Plasma Hemoglobin Using Tetramethylbenzidine (TMB). (Printed information) Fenwal Laboratories, Inc., One Baxter Parkway, Deerfield, Illinois.
3. Hanks, G.E., Cassel, M., Ray, R.N., and Chaplin, H. (1960): J. Lab. Clin. Med., 56:486-498.
4. Holland, V.R., Saunders, B.C., Rose, F.L., and Walpole, A.L. (1974): Tetrahedron, 30:3299-3302.
5. Olsson, T., Bergström, K., and Thore, A. (1981): In: Bioluminescence and Chemiluminescence: Basic chemistry and Analytical Applications, edited by M.A. DeLuca and W.D. McElroy, pp. 659-666. Academic Press, New York.
6. Schroeder, H.R., and Yeager, F.M. (1978): Anal. Chem., 50:1114-1120.
7. Standefer, J.C., and Vanderjagt, D. (1977): Clin. Chem., 23:749-751.

*Luminescent Assays: Perspectives in
Endocrinology and Clinical Chemistry*, edited by
M. Serio and M. Pazzagli, Raven Press,
New York © 1982.

Chemiluminescence Response of Polymorphonuclear Neutrophils in Diabetes Mellitus

P. De Sole, S. Lippa, G. P. Littarru, *L. Altomonte,
*G. Ghirlanda, and *A. V. Greco

*Institute of Biological Chemistry and *Department of Internal Medicine, Università Cattolica S. Cuore,
00168 Roma, Italy*

Impaired phagocytic activity of Polymorphonuclear Leukocytes (PMN-L) has long been postulated as being implicated in the well known increased susceptibility to infections in diabetic patients.

There is increasing evidence that the reported abnormality of PMN-L function in diabetes might involve defects in chemotaxis (6, 7), adherence (3), phagocytosis (2, 4, 8, 9), and the fine biochemical machinery responsible for the final events of bacterial killing (IO).

Within the various bactericidal mechanisms, the key-role of the O_2 dependent microbicidal patways is well established (I). It is generally accepted that the oxidative microbicidal activity of PMN-L is associated with the generation of electronically excited product molecules; their relaxation to the ground state, emitting photons, results in the phenomenon of Chemiluminescence (CL).

When "native" Chemiluminescence is considered, photon emission is likely to occur as the result of interaction between active intermediates of oxygen, including $O_2^{\cdot-}$, H_2O_2 and $^IO_2$, and regions of high electron density of the microbe or cellular ghosts, as found in unsaturated lipids; the products of this oxidation may be dioxetanes or other unstable molecules which disintegrate to yield electronically excited carbonyl groups capable of emitting light on relaxation to the ground state.

When "amplified" chemiluminescence is considered an oxidable substrate of high quantum yield is introduced in the system. The use of luminol (5-amino-2,3-dihydro-I,4-phtalazinedione) as an amplifier leads to an increase in CL, by approximately three orders of magnitude.

It is the aim of this paper to inquire the amplified chemiluminescence response of PMN-L from diabetic patients.

EXPERIMENTAL

Twenty patients with insulin dependent diabetes mellitus, in good metabolic control were selected for this study: 8 of these patients had a

history of recurrent infections. A group of I2 normal subjects, care-
fully screened to rule out infections, was used as control. Blood was
obtained by venipuncture, after an overnight fast, and coagulation was
prevented by the use of Heparin (Lithium salt).

PMN-L were separated from whole blood according to a modification of
the Boyum standard technique (5) i.e. a Ficoll-Hypaque density gradient
centrifugation to remove platelets and lymphocytes, followed by dextran
sedimentation and hypotonic shock for 30 seconds with NaCl 0.23% in order to remove residual red blood cells.

Isolated PMN-L were suspended in a modified Krebs-Ringer-Phosphate
medium (KRP) pH 7.4 (without $CaCl_2$ and supplemented with 0.33 mM
$Ca(NO_3)_2 \cdot 4H_2O$ and 5.5 mM glucose) to 4.0×10^5 cells/ml final concentration. To 5.0 ml of the cellular suspension 5 nmoles of luminol were added and soon after CL recorded at room temperature (22°C) with a Packard
scintillation counter, mod.2335, with the coincidence circuit inserted,
in the tritium mode. CL activity was expressed as counts per minute
(CPM). This CL obtained from PMN-L in the resting stage, before the phagocytic stimulus, will be referred as "basal chemiluminescence", and its
detection was made possible by the use of the beta-counter with the coincidence circuit inserted, which reduced the blank activity to almost
zero CPM values. Basal CL reached a peak within 4-5 min. Phagocytosis
was then inducted by addition of 0.66 mg of latex beads (Serva Feinbio-
chemia; diameter: I.I μ; latex particles/cells ratio = 500/I). An out-
burst of CL followed the addition of latex: the peak of this response,
expressed as CPM, will be mentioned as "stimulated chemiluminescence".
The ratio between stimulated CL and basal CL will be referred as Stimulation Index (S.I.).

PMN-L CHEMILUMINESCENCE PATTERN IN DIABETES MELLITUS

As shown in table I, resting CL was $0.2 \pm 0.03 \times 10^3$ CPM in normal
controls, and $2 \pm 0.3 \times 10^3$ CPM in diabetics. Conversely stimulated CL
was $780 \pm 86 \times 10^3$ CPM in normal controls, and I22.0 ± 20 in diabetic patients.

TABLE I: CHEMILUMINESCENCE RESPONSE OF GRANULOCYTES FROM NORMAL AND
DIABETIC SUBJECTS

	n	$CPM \times 10^{-3}$		S.I.
		basal CL	stimulated CL	
normal controls	12	0.2 ± 0.03	780 ± 86	3900
diabetic subjects	20	2.0 ± 0.3	122 ± 20	61
		p ∠ 0.01	p ∠ 0.01	

These data clearly show a higher basal activity together with a
lower stimulated activity in diabetics when compared to controls. This
trend is even more pronunced, within the diabetic group, for the patients
who had a history of recurrent infections, even though the difference
between these two soubgroups is significant only for what the basal CL
is concerned (table II).

TABLE II: CHEMILUMINESCENCE RESPONSE OF GRANULOCYTES FROM DIABETIC
PATIENTS

	n	basal CL	stimulated CL	C.L.
with recurrent infections	8	3.3 ± 0.5	84 ± 8.0	26
without recurrent infections	12	1.2 ± 0.3	147 ± 31	124
		$p < 0.01$	n.s.	

The behaviour of the diabetic group is very clear when one considers
the Stimulation Indexes (see table I and II). S.I. values were 3900
for the controls and 6I for the diabetic patients.

Preliminary experiments that we performed with normal PMN-L, seem to
indicate that increasing the glucose concentration in the scintillation
vial does not affect the CL response until levels of ?5 mmol/l; above
this level some inhibition occurred.

Our results are in agreement with the recent observations of Quist
and Larkins (IO) who reported a decreased stimulated glucose ocidation
and iodination by PMN-L from diabetic subjeets. The generation of reduction products of O_2, from which the oxidative bacterial killing and
the phenomenon of CL arises, is generally accepted to rely on glucose
oxidation and activation of NADPH oxidase (I).

The biochemical explanation of our findings may be related to the impaired glucose oxidation of diabetic PMN-L that we just mentioned.

From a physiological standpoint our data indicate that the neutrophil
in diabetes is somhow deficient: its persistently elevated resting activity might preclude the fully expressive response when the bacterial
challenge occurs. However this leukocyte behaviour in diabetes may be
the concequence of the high frequency of bacterial infections which ca-
rachterizes the disease and whose cause has yet to be found.

Aknowledgment: we are greatful to Mr. M. Marzialetti and M. Picarozzi
for their technical assistence in hematological counts.

REFERENCES

I. Allen, R.C. (I979): Chemiluminescence from eukaryotic and prokaryo-
   tic cells: reducing potential and oxygen requirements. Photochem.
   Photobiol., 30: I57-I63.

2. Bagdade, J.D., Root, R.K. and Bulger, R.J. (I974): Impaired lukocy-
   te function in patients with poorly controlled diabetes. Diabetes,
   23: 9-I5.

3. Bagdade, J.D., Stewart, M. and Walters, E. (I978): Impaired granulocyte adherence: a reversible defect in host defense in patients with
   poorly controlled diabetes. Diabetes, 27: 677-68I.

3. Bybee, J.D. and Rogers, D.E. (I964): The phagocytic activity of polymorphonuclear leukocytes obtained from patients with diabetes mellitus. J. Lab. Clin. Med., 64: I-I3.

5. Boyum, A. (I968): Separation of leucocytes from blood and bone marrow, with special reference to factors which influence and modify
   sedimentation properties of hematopoietic cells. Scand J. Clin. Lab.
   Invest.,2I (suppl.97): I-I09.

6. Hill, H.R., Oahn, H.D., Quie, P.G. et al. (I974): Defect in neutrophil granulocyte chemotaxis in Job's syndrome of recurrent "cold"
   Staphylococcal abscesses. Lancet, 2: 6I7-6I9.

7. Molenar, D.M., Palumbo, P.J., Wilson, W.R. and Ritts, R.E. (I976):
   Leukocytes chemotaxis in diabetic patients and their non-diabetic
   first degree relatives. Diabetes, 25: 880-883.

8. Nolan, C.M., Beaty, H.N. and Bagdade, J.D. (I978): Further characterization of the impaired bactericidal function of granulocytes in patients with poorly controlled diabetes. Diabetes, 27: 880-894.

9. Tan, J.S., Anderson J.L., Watanakunakorn, C. and Phair, J.P. (I975):
   Neutrophil function in patients with poorly controlled diabetes. Diabetes, 85: 26-33.

IO. Quist, R. and Larkins, R.G. (I98I): Decreased stimulated glucose oxi-
    dation and iodination by polymorphonuclear leukocytes from insulin-
    treated diabetic subjects. Diabetes, 30: 256-260.

Luminescent Assays: Perspectives in Endocrinology and Clinical Chemistry, edited by M. Serio and M. Pazzagli, Raven Press, New York © 1982.

Phytohemagglutinin Induced, Luminol Dependent Chemiluminescence of Peripheral Blood Leukocytes of Patients with Malignant Melanoma and Bronchial Carcinoma

S. Müller, S. Falkenberg, *Th.-M. Ernst, **U. Thalmann, M. Rühl, K. Scheider, and K.-E. Gillert

*Robert Koch-Institut des Bundesgesundheitsamtes, and *Haut- und Poliklinik der Freien Universität Berlin im Rudolf Virchow-Krankenhaus, D-1000 Berlin 65; **Städtisches Krankenhaus Heckeshorn, D-1000 Berlin 39, West Germany*

Luminol-dependent chemiluminescence (CL) measures activated oxygen compounds (O_2^-, $^1O_2$, OH·, H_2O_2) generated by stimulated immune competent cell populations (6,3). CL is applied as a measure for early events of immune competent cell activation and may be related to later events of cell differentiation, e.g. to polyclonal lymphocyte transformation (LT) as shown in a murine model of acute uremia (2).

We were interested to see if alterations of immune competent cells in cancer patients determined by LT-test could be confirmed by chemiluminescence-assay.

Leukocytes of cancer patients and healthy control donors were isolated from heparinized peripheral blood by Ficoll-Paque gradient density centrifugation (1) and their in-vitro reaction to phytohemagglutinin (PHA) was tested in the luminol-dependent CL-assay.

Additional in vitro studies with several cancer patients were performed by inducing CL in granulocytes by adding zymosan to heparinized whole blood.

12 patients with malignant melanoma, 8 in clinical stage I, 4 patients with more advanced stages, as well as 3 non radiated, non cytostatically treated, operable patients with bronchial carcinoma, were available for CL-assay. These patients were kept from groups of 35 patients with malignant melanoma in clinical stages I to III and patients with operable bronchial carcinoma of different histological types. Lymphocytes of PBL obtained by Ficoll-Paque centrifugation of peripheral whole blood were used for determining the immune status of patients by the polyclonal PHA-induced LT-test (Cells derived from bone marrow, lung lymph nodes and/or peripheral blood of 250 patients with bronchial carcinoma were tested. Data of bone marrow and lung lymph nodes are not shown.).

269

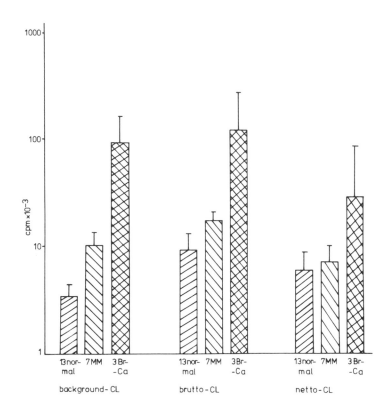

FIG. 3   PHA-induced chemiluminescence-response measured as
cpm of leukocytes derived from 7 malignant melanoma patients
(MM) (5 with clinical stage I, 2 with more advanced disease),
3 bronchial carcinoma patients (Br-Ca) and from 13 control
donors tested in parallel. For the treatment of patients see
legends of Fig. 1 and 2. CL-assay was performed according to
Fromtling et.al. (2).
Background-CL: leukocytes prior addition of PHA,
brutto-CL: CL of leukocytes after addition of PHA (20 μg /ml),
netto-CL: CL of leukocytes after addition of PHA minus background-CL. Y-axis: CL measured as the sum of cpm (divided
through 40) counted during 5 minutes.
The columns represent the mean-cpm of patients / control
donors ± SEM per group of patients / controls.

This was due to the relatively stronger increase of background-CL compared to the increase of PHA-induced CL-response in PBL of cancer patients.
Preliminary data in CL-assay performed with unfractionated
whole blood showed higher CL-background in 70% of patients
compared to the control donors (Table 2).
The results of PHA-induced, luminol dependent CL-assay in
cancer patients are characterized by 1) a non specifically
enhanced CL-activity of leukocytes prior PHA addition and

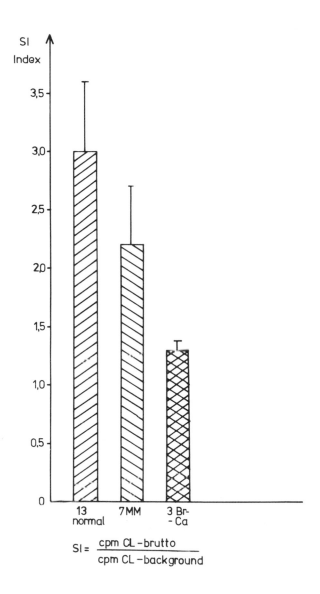

FIG. 4   CL-response expressed as stimulation index (SI) of
leukocytes derived from 7 malignant melanoma patients,
3 bronchial carcinoma patients and 13 control blood donors.
For further explanations see the legend of Fig. 3 .

TABLE 1

Chemiluminescence response to PHA[1] of Ficoll-Paque separated
leukocytes[2] of human peripheral blood inhibited by catalase,
superoxide-dismutase (SOD) and α-methyl-mannoside (α-M).

healthy blood donors		% CHEMILUMINESCENCE		
	Control	Catalase	SOD	α-M
H.H.	100	35.8	–	9.5
H.M.	100	–	–	44.5
E.L.	100	46.9	–	33.3
M.W.	100	61.4	47.6	–

[1] 20 μg/ml
[2] 2×10^6 leukocytes/ml
The concentration of catalase was 1560 U/ml,
of SOD 120 U/ml and of α-methyl-mannoside 4 mM.

TABLE 2

Background- and zymosan induced chemiluminescence in unfractionated whole blood[1] of malignant melanoma patients[2]

	7 malignant melanoma patients	5 control donors
background-CL	5,517 ± 1,068	2,667 ± 653
Zymosan[3]-induced CL	521,783 ±253,948	647,709 ± 337,371
Stimulation-index	94.5	242.8

[1] Blood was heparinized with 5 I.U. liquemine.
[2] 4 patients were in clinical stage I and 3 in advanced
disease.
[3] The zymosan-concentration was 1 mg/ml.

2) an enhanced PHA-induced CL-response compared to control
donors.
Corresponding altered CL-activity is found in granulocytes
when assayed in the whole blood model.
Since it is known that cancer patients' acessory cells as
macrophages exhibit enhanced killer cell activity (5) and
an increase of %-adherence to a solid surface (4), the altered CL-levels found in leukocytes of patients as presented here may indicate altered acessory cell function.
Therefore it seems to be presumable that CL-assay could
serve as another parameter for measuring acessory cell dysfunction in cancer patients.
Although characteristic changes in leukocyte functions are
expressed by both assays, a significant correlation between
the results of the LT-test and the CL-assay in the tested
cancer patients can not be seen.

ACKNOWLEDGEMENTS

This work was supported by the Umweltbundesamt Berlin and
the Georg and Agnes Blumenthal-Stiftung. We thank Dr. Gabler
for kindly providing us cells and clinical data from bronchial carcinoma patients.

REFERENCES

1. Bøyum, A. (1968): Scand. J. Clin. Invest., Suppl 97: 21
2. Fromtling, R.A., Fromtling, A.M., Staib, F., and Müller,
   S. (1981): Infect. Immun., 32: 1073-1078
3. Kato, T., Wokalek, H., Schöpf, E., Eggert, H., Ernst, M.,
   Rietschel, E. Th., and Fischer, H. (1981): Klin. Wochen-
   schr., 59: 203-211
4. Müller, S., and Ernst, Th.-M. (1980): Arch. Dermatol. Res.,
   268: 167-181
5. Nyholm, R.F., and Currie, G.A. (1978): Br. J. Cancer, 37:
   337-334
6. Wrogemann, K., Weidemann, M.J., Ketelsen, U.-P., Weckerle,
   H., and Fischer, H. (1980): Europ. J. Immunol., 10: 36-40

Subject Index

Subject Index

Acridinium ester labelled IgG, 151–153

Acridinium esters, 148, 187; *see also* Estradiol, acridinium ester of

Active oxygens, *see* Oxygens, active

Adenine nucleotides, in spermatozoa, 79–86
  variation in, 81, 84

Adenylates, 67–68

Adipose tissue, human versus other species, 56

ADP
  preparations of, 35
  in spermatozoa, 79–86
  variation of, 81, 84

Adrenaline, 221–226
  oxidation rate, noradrenaline versus, 223–224

Aequora, substrate in, 3

Alcohol dehydrogenase concentrations, 116

Aldehyde
  in bacterial luminescence, 97–98
  chemical structure of, 3

Alloxan, 218

Alpha-fetoprotein (AFP), antibodies to, 153

Aminochrome pathway, catecholamine oxidation and, 226

4-Aminophtalhydrazide, *see* Isoluminol

Androsterone, light intensity and, 117, 118

Antibiotics, 96
  short term tests for bacterial, 99–101

Antibodies
  to alpha-fetoprotein (AFP), 153
  chemiluminescence labelled, 147–154; *see also* Antibody-enhanced chemiluminesce; Immunoassays, chemiluminescent
  advantages of, 148, 154
  preparation of, 150–151

Antibody-enhanced chemiluminescence
  antibody role in, 196–197
  definition of, 191
  parameters of, 198
  of progesterone, 191–198

Anti-human IgG, 140–141
  CIA for, 139

Antimicrobial agents, 96

Antioxidants, 215

Arthropod, substrates in, 3

Ascorbic acid, 216–217

ATP, 4–5; *see also specific ATP listings*
  converting reactions, 32–34
  red blood cell viability and levels of, 12

ATP/ADP ratio, 81, 84

ATP bioluminescence assay, 5–7, 36–37
  bacterial, 12–13
  purified reagents with stable light emission in, 35
  sperm antibodies, determination of, 89–93
  in spermatozoa, human, 79–86
  variation of, 81, 84
  with firefly luciferase, 39–42
  application of, 36–42
  ATP degrading enzymes and, 39–40
  cell lysis and, 41
  electron transport linked phosphorylation and, 41
  end point assays of metabolites, 37–39
  enzymes, kinetic assays of, 39–40
  firefly luciferase reaction in, 39–40
  immunoassays, 41–42
  instrumentation for, 36
  light emission, kinetics of, 32–34, 47–51
  metabolites, kinetic assays of, 39–40
  reagents for, 34–35

ATP degrading enzymes, ATP